Surgical Anatomy of the Orbit

C.A.Luce

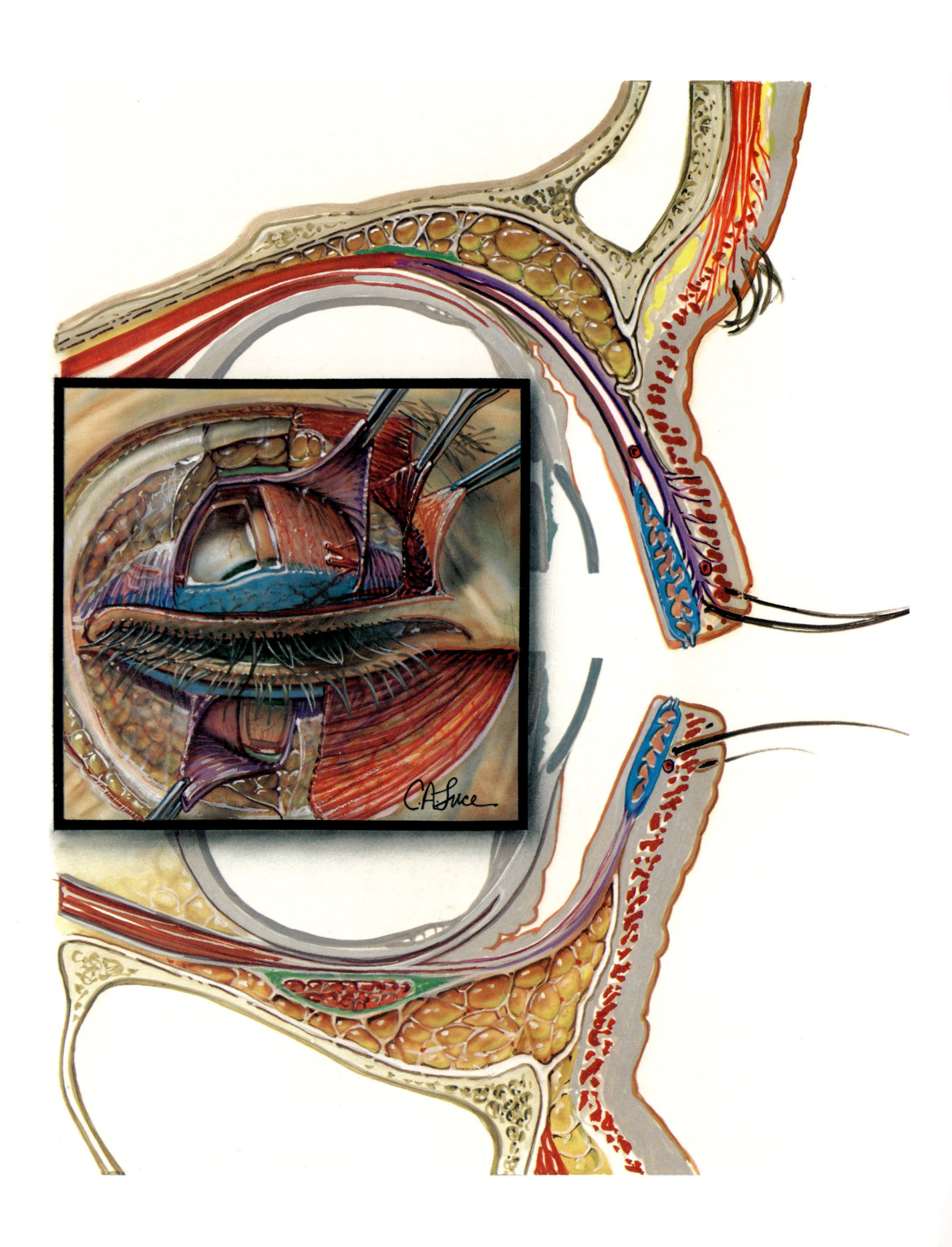

Surgical Anatomy of the Orbit

Barry M. Zide, M.D., D.M.D.
Assistant Professor of Plastic Surgery
New York University Medical Center
Bellevue Hospital Center
Manhattan Eye, Ear, and Throat Hospital
Manhattan Veterans Administration Hospital
Attending Staff
New York Eye and Ear Infirmary
New York, New York

Glenn W. Jelks, M.D.
Assistant Professor of Plastic Surgery
New York University Medical Center
Bellevue Hospital Center
Manhattan Eye, Ear, and Throat Hospital
Manhattan Veterans Administration Hospital
Attending Staff
New York Eye and Ear Infirmary
New York, New York

Illustrator
Craig Luce, M.S.

Raven Press ■ New York

Raven Press, 1185 Avenue of the Americas, New York, New York 10036

©1985 by Raven Press Books, Ltd. All rights reserved. This book is protected by copyright. No part of it may be reproduced, stored in a retrieval system, or transmitted, in any form or by any means, electronic, mechanical, photocopying, recording, or otherwise, without the prior written permission of the publisher.

Made in the United States of America

Figures 3-6A and 3-15 are reproduced from *Clinics in Plastic Surgery*, 1981, Vol. 8, No. 4, with permission.

Figures 2-15, 3-13, 3-16, 3-17 A & B, 3-21 A & B, 6-5 A & B, and 8-8A are reproduced from *Plastic and Reconstructive Surgery*, Vol. 74, No. 2, with permission.

Figure 5-4 is reproduced from *Annals of Plastic Surgery*, with permission.

Library of Congress Cataloging-in-Publication Data

Zide, Barry M.
    Surgical anatomy of the orbit.

    Includes bibliographies and index.
    1. Eye-sockets—Anatomy.   2. Anatomy, Surgical and topographical.
  I. Jelks, Glenn W.   II. Title.
[DNLM: 1. Orbit—anatomy & histology. 2. Orbit—surgery. WW 202 Z64s]
QM511.Z53   1985   611'.84   83—42619
ISBN 0-88167—054—5

The material contained in this volume was submitted as previously unpublished material, except in the instances in which credit has been given to the source from which some of the illustrative material was derived.
Great care has been taken to maintain the accuracy of the information contained in the volume. However, Raven Press cannot be held responsible for errors or for any consequences arising from the use of the information contained herein.

Production editor and book design   Anne G. Friedman

Printed in Hong Kong

*To our wives, Ellen and Liz,
whose support was everpresent*

Preface

The expansion of surgical techniques within the last decade demands that the surgeon maximize his anatomical knowledge in conjunction with his surgical skills. Craniofacial deformities, trauma, or extirpative requirements compel a cooperative effort among multiple surgical specialists including ophthalmologists, plastic surgeons, neurosurgeons, otolaryngologists, and maxillofacial surgeons. The eye and orbit represent a major crossroads of surgical anatomic dissection.

This text, targeted for the clinical surgeon, allows a trial run the night before an operation. How often has the reader ruminated about a procedure that might have gone more predictably with the benefit of a preliminary dissection, or hesitated to apply a new technique because of unfamiliarity? Surgeons have been frustrated after hours of rummaging through stacks of texts with verbose discussions of poorly illustrated and complexly labeled drawings that provide little assistance for the operating theater.

The artist's renderings are designed to complement the fresh dissections and to further the understanding of the complex eyelid and orbital anatomy. Labeling of diagrams has been minimized except when necessary to present an overview as has been done in Chapter 1 for the nerves and arteries of the orbit. The reader can scan the material rapidly or review it slowly multiple times with ease.

The specimens used for this book were usually between 12 and 48 hours postmortem. Multiple specimens were used for short periods (less than two hours) to provide a fresh, bloodless field. Furthermore, smaller dissections performed in isolation did not suffer from the confusion that occurs when other dissected tissues are adjacent to the area of demonstration.

The authors met in 1979 when Barry Zide was starting his craniofacial fellowship with Joseph G. McCarthy, while Glenn Jelks was a senior resident in plastic surgery at NYU Medical Center, but already a fully trained ophthalmologist. We both felt that a clear understanding of orbital anatomy was a prerequisite for maturation as a craniofacial or ophthalmologic plastic surgeon. Subsequently, Barry Zide joined the faculty at the University of Virginia where Craig Luce was producing high quality art for the department of ophthalmology. His superb work, so evident here, forms the backbone of this atlas since understanding orbital anatomy demands a 3-dimensional conceptualization which can only be conveyed by such a gifted artist. One need only peruse Chapter 8 on the fascial structures of the orbit to obtain an understanding of a topic hitherto nebulous for many orbital surgeons. The diagrams of the eyelids and lateral retinaculum when used in conjunction with the dissections will provide guidance for the reader engaged in orbital surgery. Although this atlas was not intended as a dissection manual, it may be extremely helpful during formal laboratory study.

This book reflects the authors' personal philosophy. We realized during our preparations that an exhaustive bibliography would be counterproductive. We have reviewed a great deal of reference material which has been distilled into this tome. The major texts from which this specific information was provided are noted below.

We have learned a great deal in preparing this text and hope that you will find it valuable in your practice.

Barry M. Zide
Glenn W. Jelks

Bibliography

Beard, C., and Quickert, M. (1977): *Anatomy of the Orbit*, 2nd edit. Aesculapius, Birmingham.
Doxanas, M. T., and Anderson, R. L. (1984): *Clinical Orbital Anatomy*. Williams and Wilkins, Baltimore.
Duker-Elder, S. (1961): *The Anatomy of the Visual System*. System of Ophthalmology Series, Vol. 2. C. V. Mosby, St. Louis.
Hollingshead, W. H. (1982): *Anatomy for Surgeons*, Vol. 1. *The Head and Neck*, 3rd edit. Harper and Row, Philadelphia.
Lang, J. (1983): *Clinical Anatomy of the Head*. Springer Verlag, Berlin, NewYork.
Warwick, R. (1976): *Eugene Wolff's Anatomy of the Eye and Orbit*, 7th edit. W. B. Saunders, Great Britain.

Contents

Preface		*vii*
Foreword		*xi*
1.	Bones, Vessels, and Nerves	1
2.	Forehead, Temporal Region, and Cheek	13
3.	The Eyelids	21
4.	Lacrimal Apparatus	33
5.	Medial Canthus	41
6.	Lateral Retinaculum	47
7.	Orbital Dissection	51
8.	Extraocular Muscles and Associated Fascial Structures	59
9.	Intracranial Dissection	67
	Subject Index	73

Foreword

The development of modern medicine has paralleled the history of anatomical studies. According to Galen, Herophilus (approximately 300 B.C.) was the first person to dissect both humans and animals for learning purposes. Galen (129–199 A.D.) continued this tradition with a sixteen-book treatise, *On Anatomical Procedure*. His theories of physiology persisted until Harvey and his anatomical studies were inherited by Vesalius thirteen centuries later.

Vesalius, born in Brussels in 1514, received a Galenic training at the Universities of Louvain and Paris. His *Fabrica* was published in 1543 while he was a professor at Padua. Anatomy immediately changed from a Galenic to a Vesalian discipline with this publication. In the 7th book of the *Fabrica,* he described the eye, but made several erroneous and inadequate descriptions, and offered no discussion of the adnexal structures.

By the time the authors were students—approximately four centuries later—there existed an attitude among medical faculties that everything known about the anatomy of the human body was described by Vesalius or "the Germans in the 19th Century." At this time the study of anatomy had been relegated to a small portion of the medical school curriculum. Medical science had shifted from the pedagogic emphasis of gross anatomy to the molecular confines of the cell.

The advances in reconstructive plastic surgery in the last fifteen years have demonstrated the fallacy of this attitude. New anatomical studies, usually initiated by clinical surgeons, of the skin circulation, internal structure of nerves, blood supply of the muscles, craniofacial skeleton, and finally the intricacies of the periorbital area, have had a profound effect on the proliferation of many new techniques—a true renaissance in reconstructive plastic surgery.

Doctors Zide and Jelks, united by a keen interest in orbital anatomy, bring a diverse background to their collaborative effort. The former approached his plastic surgery career through dentistry and general surgery, the latter through ophthalmology. Drawn to reconstructive plastic surgery of the periorbital region, they quickly realized the limitations of existing anatomical concepts of this region, and thus began an anatomical odyssey of the orbital region.

In this text, the fine structures of the periorbital area have been illustrated with the clarity and elegance which only modern printing techniques permit. As a first step, anatomical studies were done on human cadavers with painstaking care and then documented by photographs. The latter are beautifully complemented by the watercolors of a master artist, Craig Luce.

The reader will benefit immensely from these efforts. In a single volume, one will

FOREWORD

have immediate access to the multilayered intricacies of the eyelids, the geometric compartmentalization of the orbital contents, and the complexities of the nasolacrimal apparatus. With increased knowledge of orbital anatomy, it is inevitable that the field of ophthalmic plastic surgery will move forward to solve many of the current clinical problems.

Joseph G. McCarthy
Lawrence D. Bell, Professor
of Plastic Surgery
New York University

1

Bones, Vessels, and Nerves

The ocular globes reside in two symmetrical bony cavities called the orbits. Seven bones contribute to form the orbital walls. The classic description of the shape of the orbit is that of a four-sided pyramid with its base directed anteriorly. Actually, the orbit is quite pear shaped, with its widest diameter approximately 1 cm within the orbital rim.

The orbit must be considered a complex entity in relation to its surrounding and associated structures. Nerves and vessels enter the orbit, and their course and distribution must be understood. The aerated sinuses as well as the anterior and middle cranial fossae are intimately related to the orbital walls.

Note to the reader: Throughout this book, all dissections will be presented using the *right* orbit.

Chapter 1

FIG. 1-1. Bony components of the right orbit *(colored):* (1) maxilla *(orange)*; (2) zygoma *(beige)*; (3) sphenoid bone, greater wing *(light blue)*; lesser wing *(dark blue)*; (4) palatine bone *(light green)*; (5) ethmoid bone *(purple)*; (6) lacrimal bone *(pink)*; (7) frontal bone *(green)*.

FIG. 1-2. Lateral oblique right orbit.

Bones, Vessels, and Nerves

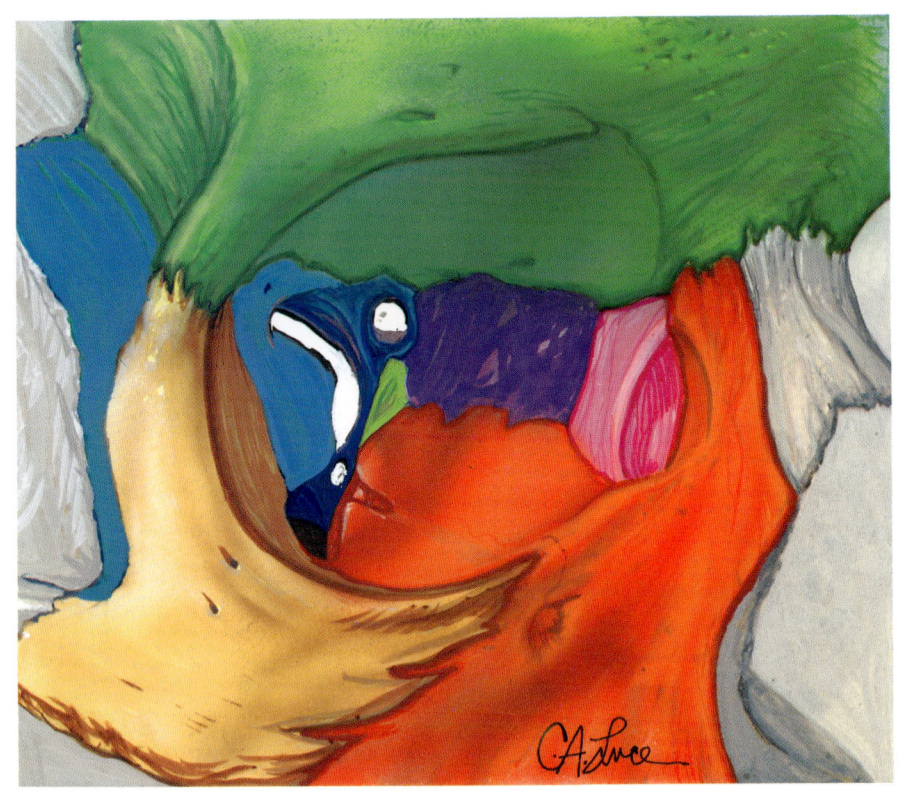

Fig. 1-1.

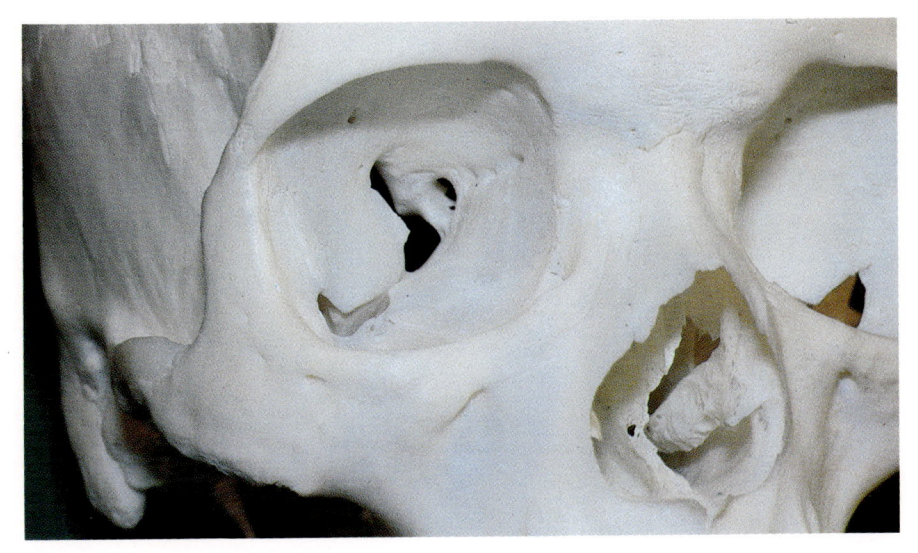

Fig. 1-2.

Chapter 1

FIG. 1-3. The walls. **A:** The roof. This wall is composed mainly of the orbital plate of the frontal bone. Posteriorly, it receives a minor contribution from the lesser wing of the sphenoid bone.

Located within the anterolateral portion of the roof, note a smooth, wide depression for the lacrimal gland, the lacrimal fossa (LF). Approximately 5 mm posterior to the medial aspect of the rim, the trochlear fossa (TF) denotes the attachment of the cartilaginous pulley for the tendon of the superior oblique muscle. The triangular roof narrows as it proceeds toward the apex, where a vertically oval opening, the optic foramen (OF), marks the orbital end of the optic canal.

B: The lateral wall. The lateral wall is formed primarily by the orbital surface of the zygomatic bone (Z) and the greater wing of the sphenoid bone (S). The sphenoid portion of the lateral wall is separated from the roof by the superior orbital fissure (SOF) and from the floor by the inferior orbital fissure (IOF).

A small bony promontory may be noted just within the orbital rim. This important landmark, Whitnall's tubercle (WT), is the point of attachment for several structures to be described later. At the anterior end of the inferior orbital fissure, a small groove may be noted for the passage of the zygomatic nerve and vessels *(arrow)*. The groove often develops into a canal that divides within bone to conduct the zygomaticofacial vessels and nerves onto the face and the zygomaticotemporal vessels and nerves into the temporal fossa. The zygomaticofacial and zygomaticotemporal complexes may pass through separate foramina (ZF).

Near the upper end of the superior orbital fissure, the orbital branch of the middle meningeal artery may pass through the meningeal foramen (MF).

The inferior orbital fissure separates the greater sphenoid wing portion of the lateral wall from the floor. Posteriorly, the foramen rotundum (FR) may be seen, whereas more anteriorly, the fissure communicates with the pterygopalatine fossa as well as the infratemporal fossa. Through this fissure pass 1) the maxillary division of the trigeminal nerve, V_2, and its branches; the 2) infraorbital artery; 3) branches of the sphenopalatine ganglion; and 4) branches of the inferior ophthalmic vein to the pterygoid plexus.

C: The floor. The thin orbital floor is composed of the orbital plate of the maxilla, the zygomatic bone anterolaterally, and the orbital process of the palatine bone posteriorly. A shallow rough area at the anteromedial angle *(stippled)* marks the origin of the inferior oblique muscle. The infraorbital groove (IG) runs forward from the inferior orbital fissure. Anteriorly, the groove becomes a canal within the maxilla, finally forming the infraorbital foramen on the face of the maxilla. The groove and canal transmit the infraorbital nerve and artery. From the lower aspect of this nerve, middle superior alveolar nerves (occasionally) emanate to supply the bicuspid teeth. More anteriorly and 5–20mm prior to the infraorbital nerve exit from its foramen, the anterior superior alveolar nerves descend medially along the inner face of the maxilla or within a canal to supply sensation to the anterior three teeth and gingiva.

D: The medial wall. The medial wall is quadrangular in shape and is composed of four bones: 1) the ethmoid bone centrally; 2) the frontal bone superoanteriorly; 3) the lacrimal bone inferoanteriorly; and 4) the sphenoid bone posteriorly. The inferior orbital margin continues upward into the anterior lacrimal crest (ALC), part of the frontal process of the maxilla. The superomedial margin continues downward into the posterior lacrimal crest (PLC) part of the lacrimal bone. Between these rests the fossa for the lacrimal sac. Usually, the fossa is approximately 14 mm in height.

The medial wall is quite thin, and the ethmoidal portion has been termed lamina papyracea. The anterior and posterior ethmoidal foramina (AE, PE) are noted at the frontoethmoidal suture and denote the level of the cribriform plate. The anterior ethmoidal foramen transmits the anterior ethmoidal artery and the anterior ethmoidal nerve branches of the nasociliary nerve. The posterior ethmoidal foramen provides a passage for the posterior ethmoidal artery and, occasionally, for a sphenoethmoidal nerve branch from the nasociliary nerve.

Bones, Vessels, and Nerves

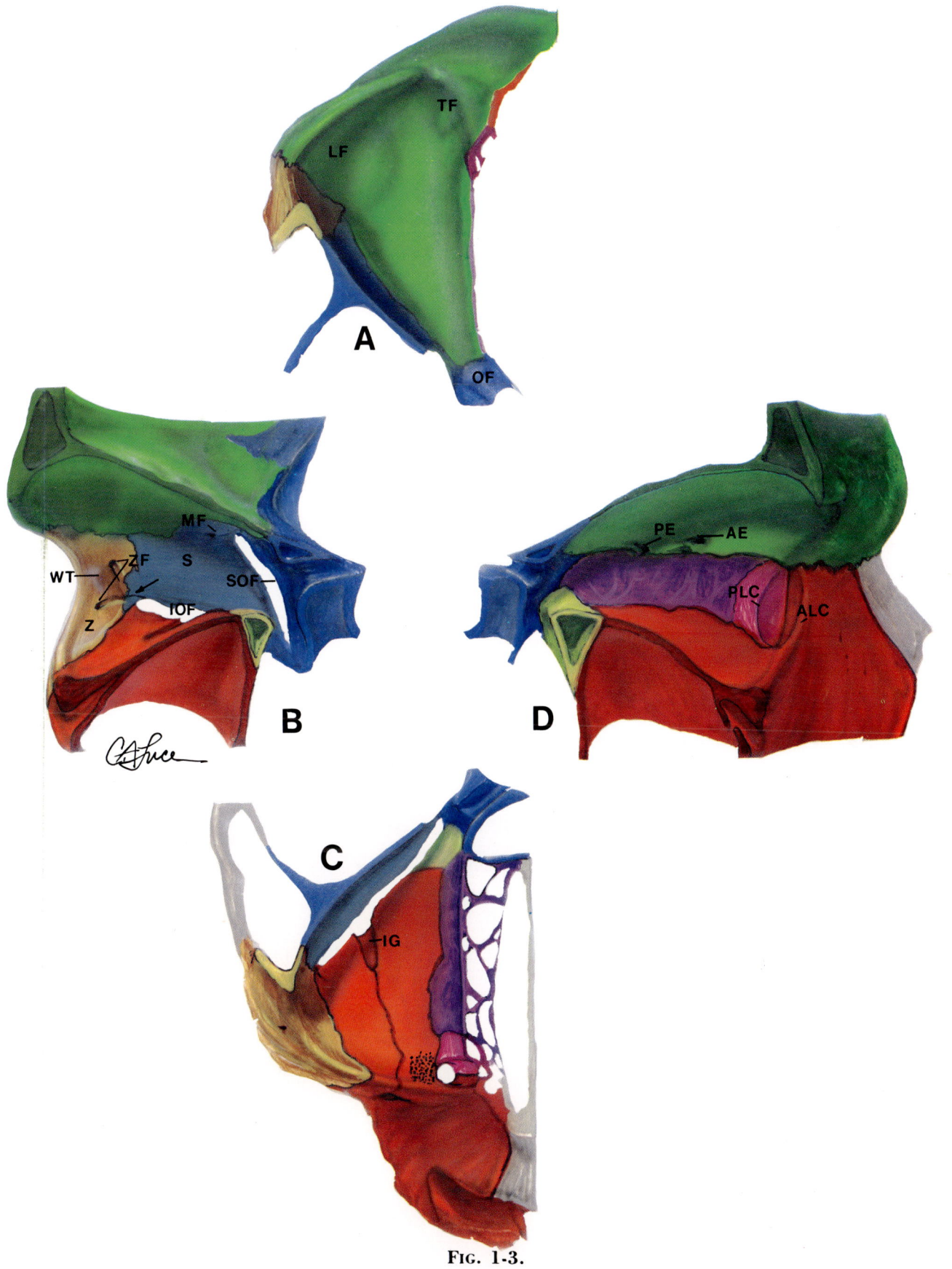

Fig. 1-3.

5

CHAPTER 1

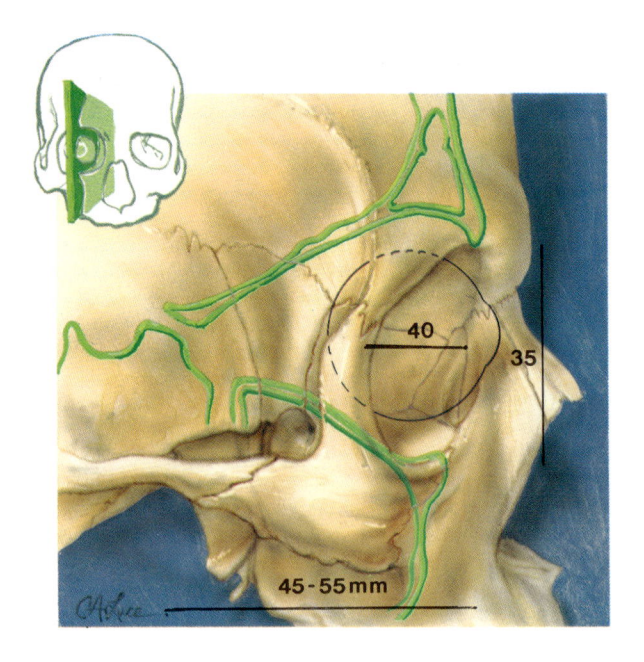

FIG. 1-4. Orbital *height* at the entrance measures approximately *35 mm*, as opposed to a usual adult width of 40 mm. Orbital depth measured to the optic strut (the bone between the optic foramen and the superior orbital fissure) varies from 45 to 55 mm.

FIG. 1-5. Only the lacrimal bone (L) exists wholly within the orbital confines. Note how the frontal bone slopes back to join the frontal process of the zygoma at the zygomaticofrontal suture *(arrow)*. The temporal fossa lies behind the zygomatic bone (Z). The foramen for the zygomaticofacial nerve (ZF) varies greatly in position on the anterior prominence of the zygomatic bone.

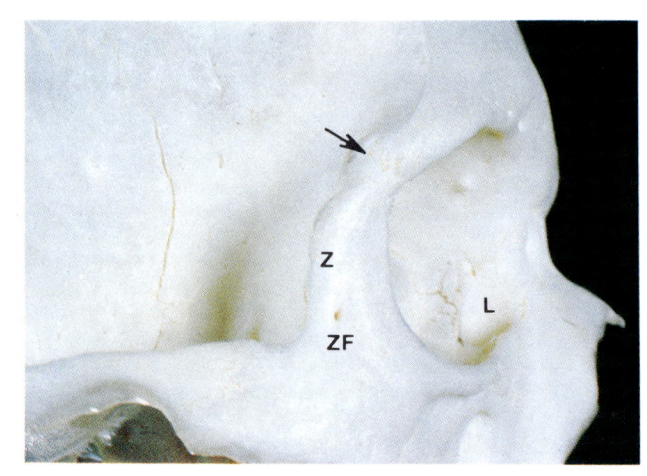

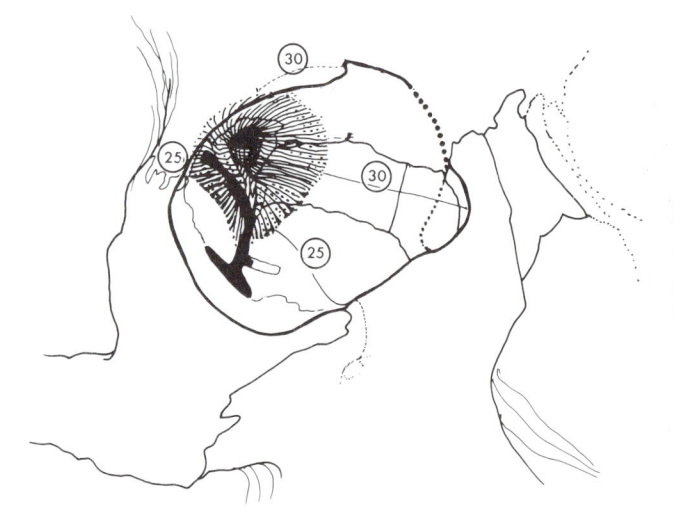

FIG. 1-6. The safe distances for dissection along each wall are noted in millimeters. The danger zone is shaded posteriorly. Deeper safe subperiosteal dissection may be performed medially or superiorly.

BONES, VESSELS, AND NERVES

FIG. 1-7. The angle between the lateral walls of both orbits is approximately 90°. The angle between the lateral and medial walls of a single side is approximately 45°. The two medial walls appear almost parallel. The orbital axis (OX) and visual axis (VX) do not coincide but diverge at an angle of approximately 23°. The orbital axis is the bisection line between the medial and lateral walls. The visual axis corresponds to the position of the eye in straight gaze.

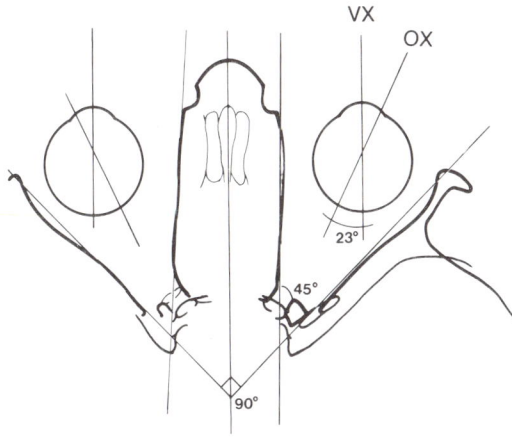

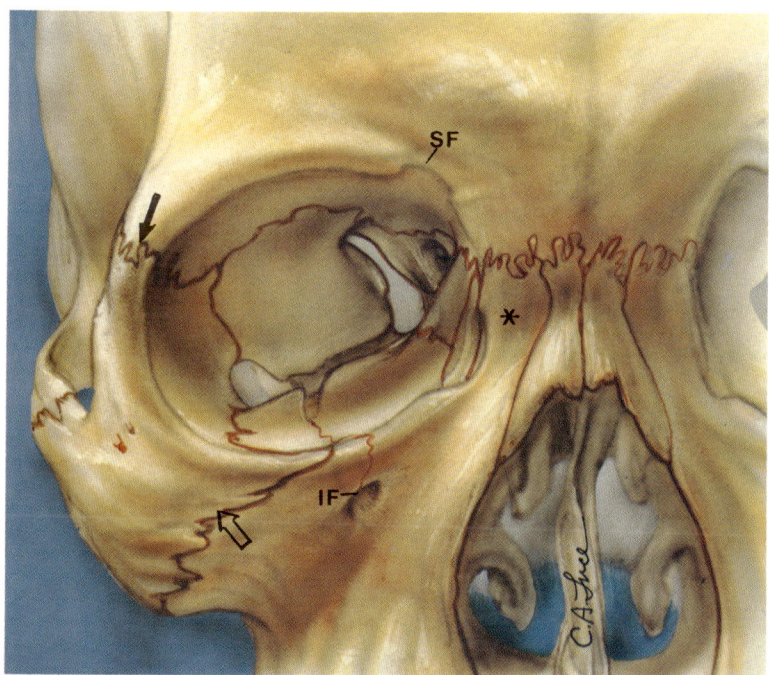

FIG. 1-8. The infraorbital foramen (IF) is approximately 4 mm in diameter and may be found approximately 7 mm ± 4 mm from the infraorbital rim. The frontal process of the maxilla (*) extends upward to form part of the lateral wall of the nose. The zygoma articulates with the maxilla at the zygomatomaxillary suture *(open arrow)*. On either side of the glabella (midforehead), the frontal bone is somewhat prominent, forming the supraciliary arches that lie just above the upper orbital margins. The zygomatic process of the frontal bone extends laterally to articulate with the frontal process of the zygoma at the zygomaticofrontal suture *(solid arrow)*. The supraorbital notch, less commonly a foramen (SF), is noted at the medial aspect of the superior orbital rim.

FIG. 1-9. The keystone to the bony orbit is the sphenoid bone shown here from its anterior aspect. All neurovascular structures to the orbit pass through this bone. The superior orbital fissure (*) is the gap between the lesser wing *(dark blue)* and the greater wing *(light blue)* of the sphenoid bone. The optic canal is medial to the superior orbital fissure within the substance of the lesser wing.

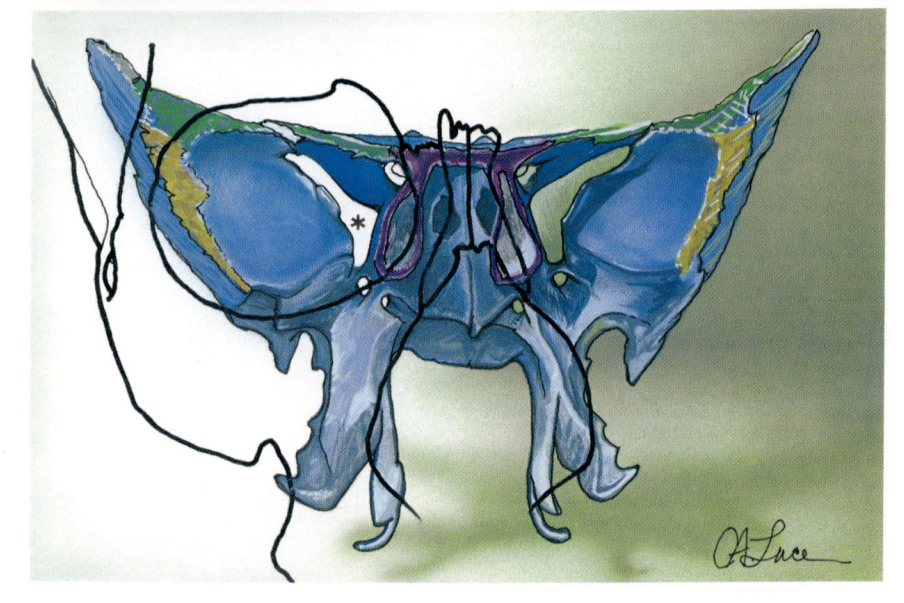

7

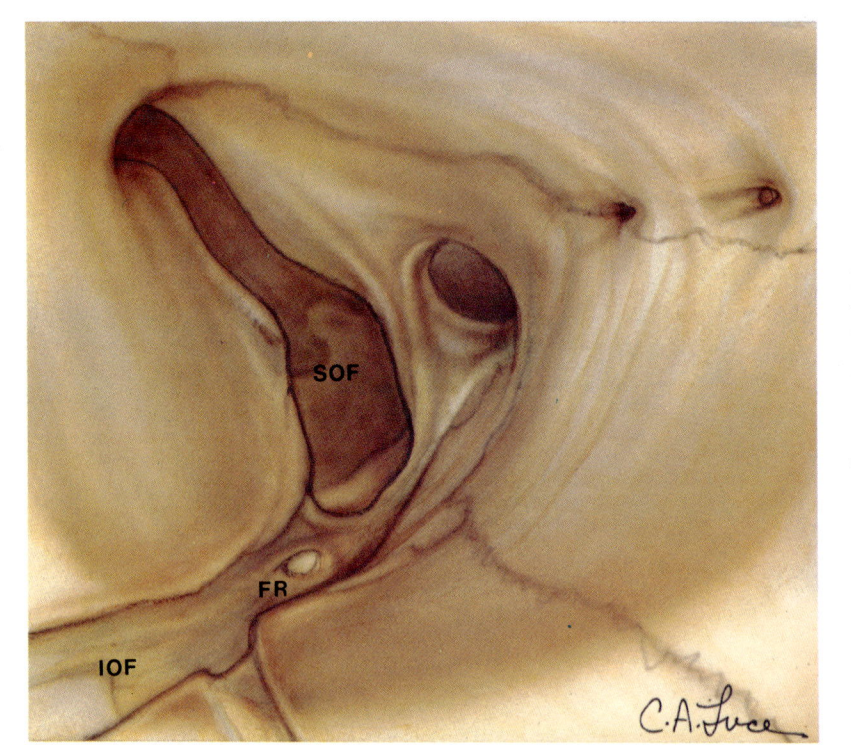

Fig. 1-10. The superior orbital fissure widens medially where it lies below the level of the optic foramen. Note the foramen rotundum (FR) just inferior to the confluence between the superior orbital fissure and inferior orbital fissure (IOF). The total length of the superior orbital fissure is 22 mm.

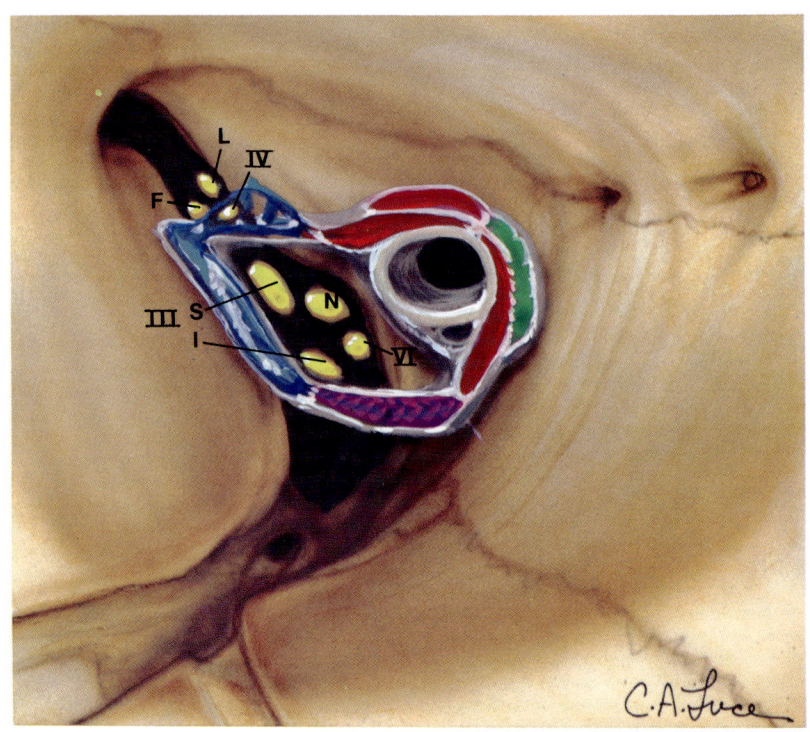

Fig. 1-11. The common tendinous ring, or annulus of Zinn, divides the superior orbital fissure. The extraocular muscles arise from this common ring. The portion of the annulus that is formed by the origin of the lateral rectus muscle *(blue)* divides the superior orbital fissure into two compartments. That area encircled by the annulus is termed the *oculomotor foramen,* which opens into the middle cranial fossa and transmits (1) cranial nerve III (upper and lower divisions); (2) cranial nerve VI; (3) the nasociliary branch of cranial nerve V; (4) ophthalmic veins; (5) the orbital branch of the middle meningeal artery (occasionally); and (6) sympathetic nerve fibers. Above the annulus note the trochlear nerve (IV) and the frontal and lacrimal branches of cranial nerve V. It is important to realize that the frontal and lacrimal branches of the ophthalmic division of cranial nerve V and the trochlear nerve enter the orbit outside the muscle cone.

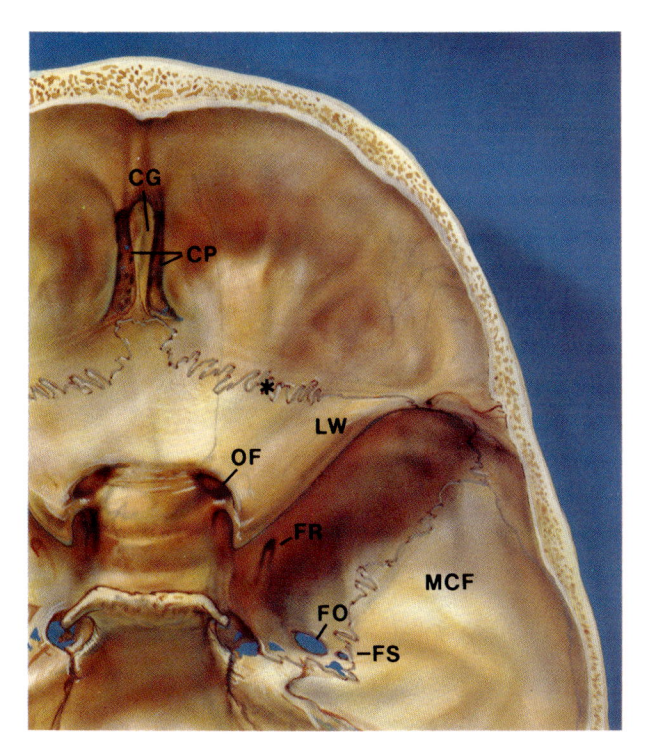

Fig. 1-12. The skullcap is removed to expose the roof of the right orbit. For orientation, note the crista galli (CG), straddled by paired cribriform plates (CP). The optic foramen (OF) may be seen within the lesser wing of the sphenoid bone (LW). The frontosphenoidal sutures (*) separate frontal bone from the more posterior sphenoid bone. The foramen rotundum (FR), foramen spinosum (FS), and foramen ovale (FO) are noted within the middle cranial fossa (MCF).

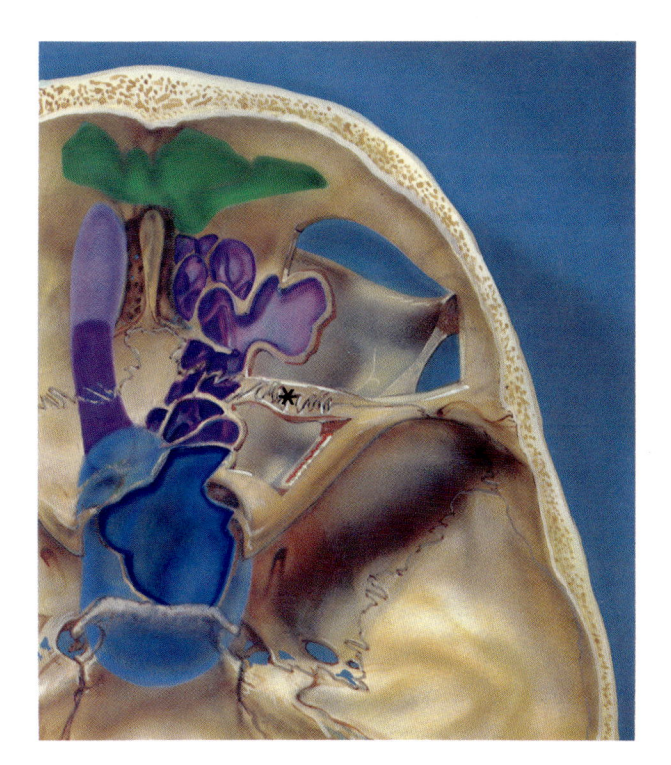

Fig. 1-13. The roof of the orbit is removed except for the frontosphenoid suture (*). The sinuses are marked as follows: frontal sinus *(green)*; anterior ethmoidal air cells *(light purple)*; posterior ethmoidal air cells *(dark purple)*; and sphenoid sinus *(blue)*.

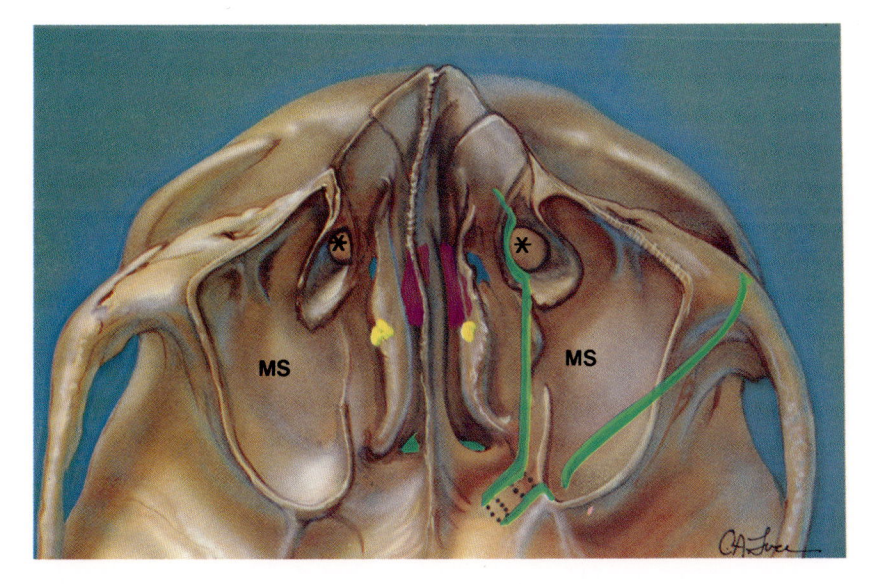

Fig. 1-14. The maxillary sinuses (MS) are exposed after transverse section below the orbits. The orbital walls are outlined *(green)*. The transected nasolacrimal canals (*), which later empty into the inferior meati, are noted medially on each side. The nasofrontal ducts *(blue)* empty into the anterior portion of the middle meati most commonly. The ethmoidal ostia *(yellow)* usually enter the nose in the middle meatus at its midportion. The sphenoid sinuses empty into the nose at the sphenoethmoid recesses *(green)*. The relative position of the cribriform plate is noted *(magenta)*.

CHAPTER 1

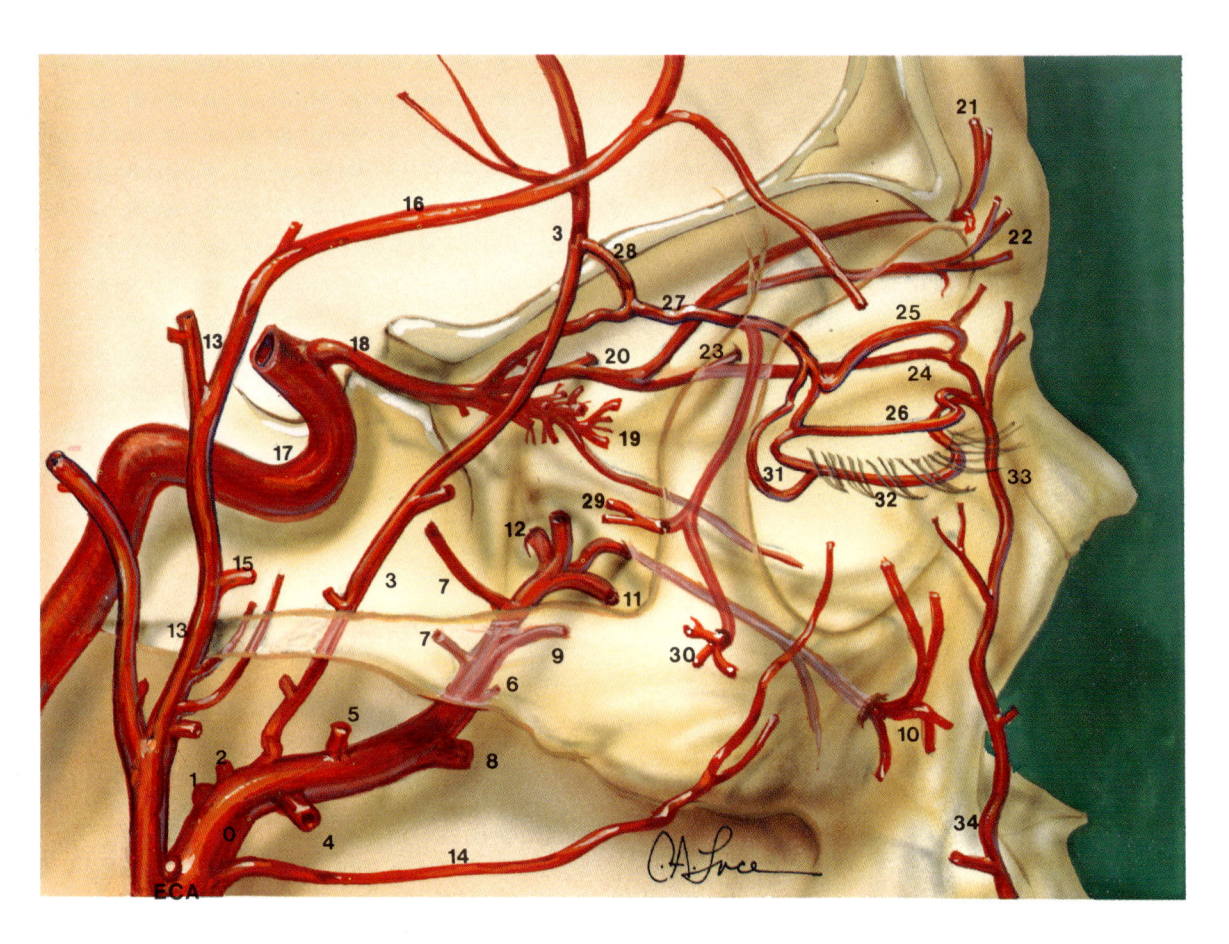

FIG. 1-15. The relationship of the internal and external carotid arterial systems to the orbit. **A:** Lateral view: The two terminal branches of the external carotid artery are the internal maxillary artery and superficial temporal artery.

FIG. 1-15. **A:** Internal maxillary artery (O):

(1) deep auricular;
(2) anterior tympanic;
(3) middle meningeal;
(4) inferior alveolar;
(5) masseteric;
(6) pterygoid;
(7) deep temporal;
(8) buccal;
(9) posterior superior alveolar;
(10) infraorbital;
(11) sphenopalatine;
(12) artery of the pterygoid canal;
(13) superficial temporal artery;
(14) transverse facial;
(15) zygomatico-orbital;
(16) frontal branch;
(17) internal carotid artery;
(18) ophthalmic;
(19) intraconal branches of ophthalmic artery (see Fig. 1-15B);
(20) posterior ethmoidal branch of ophthalmic;
(21) supraorbital artery;
(22) supratrochlear;
(23) anterior ethmoidal branch of ophthalmic;
(24) infratrochlear;
(25) peripheral arcade (superior);
(26) marginal arcade (superior);
(27) lacrimal;
(28) recurrent meningeal;
(29) zygomaticotemporal;
(30) zygomaticofacial;
(31) lateral palpebral;
(32) inferior marginal arcade;
(33) angular;
(34) facial;
(35) central retinal;
(36) lateral posterior ciliary;
(37) muscular branches to superior rectus, to levator palpebrae, and to superior oblique;
(38) medial posterior ciliary;
(39) short ciliary;
(40) long ciliary;
(41) anterior ciliary;
(42) greater circle of iris;
(43) lesser circle of iris;
(44) episcleral;
(45) subconjunctival;
(46) conjunctival;
(47) marginal arcade;
(48) vortex vein;
(49) medial palpebral;
(50) dorsal nasal.

10

BONES, VESSELS, AND NERVES

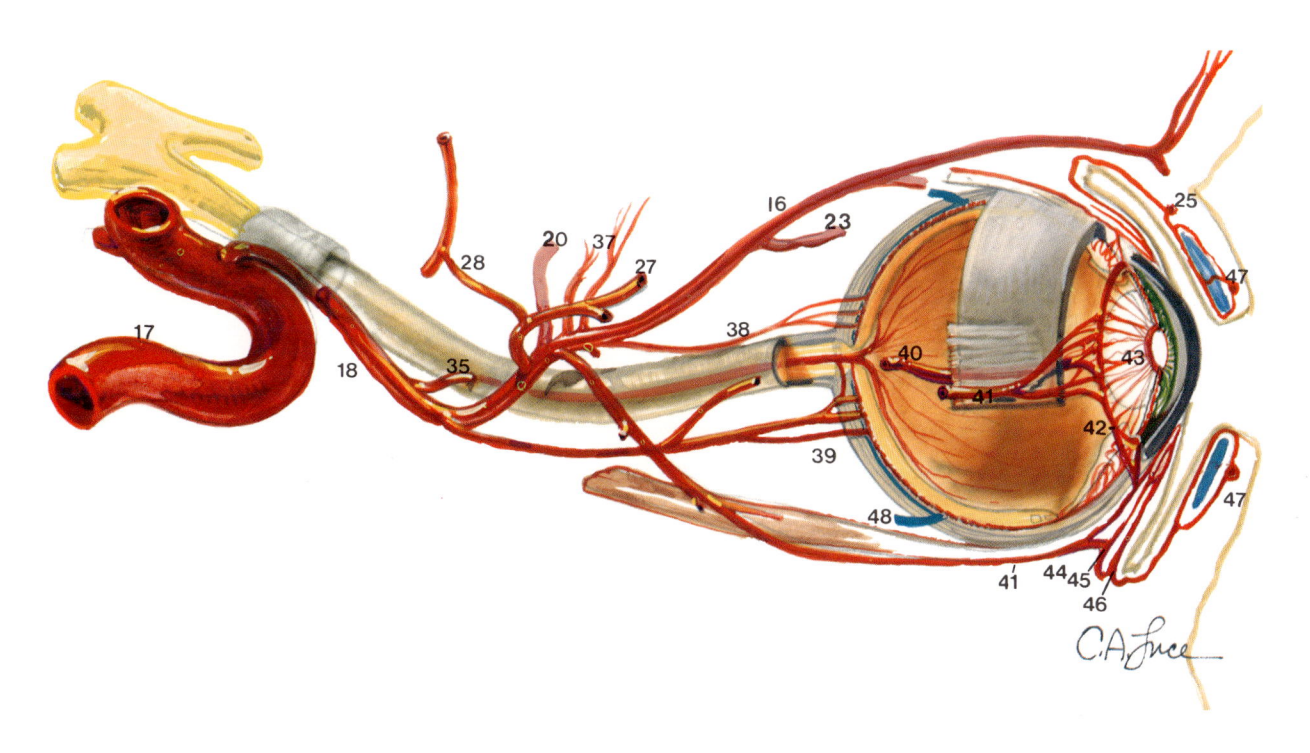

FIG. 1-15. B: The ophthalmic artery in the muscle cone.

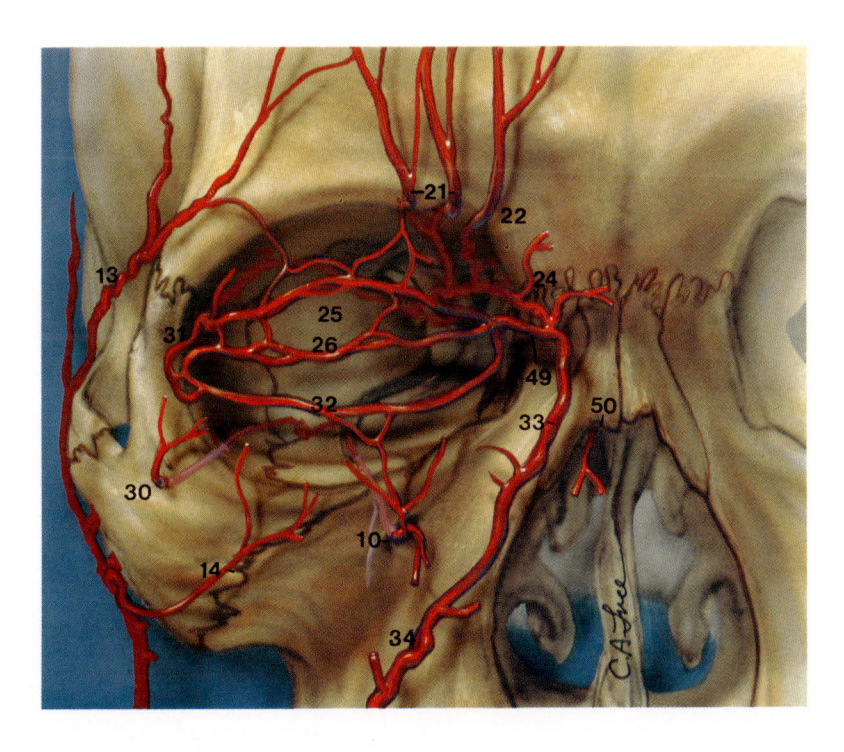

FIG. 1-15. C: The main points here are the following: First, most branches of the ophthalmic artery stem from the posterior third of the orbit to travel forward. Second, the ophthalmic artery is tethered to the medial orbital wall by the ethmoid arteries. Third, the collateralization that occurs among ICA (17), the recurrent meningeal (28), and the facial arterial tree (33, 34) accounts for reversal of flow when the ICA is obstructed. Finally, the central retinal artery enters the optic nerve in the posterior third.

11

Chapter 1

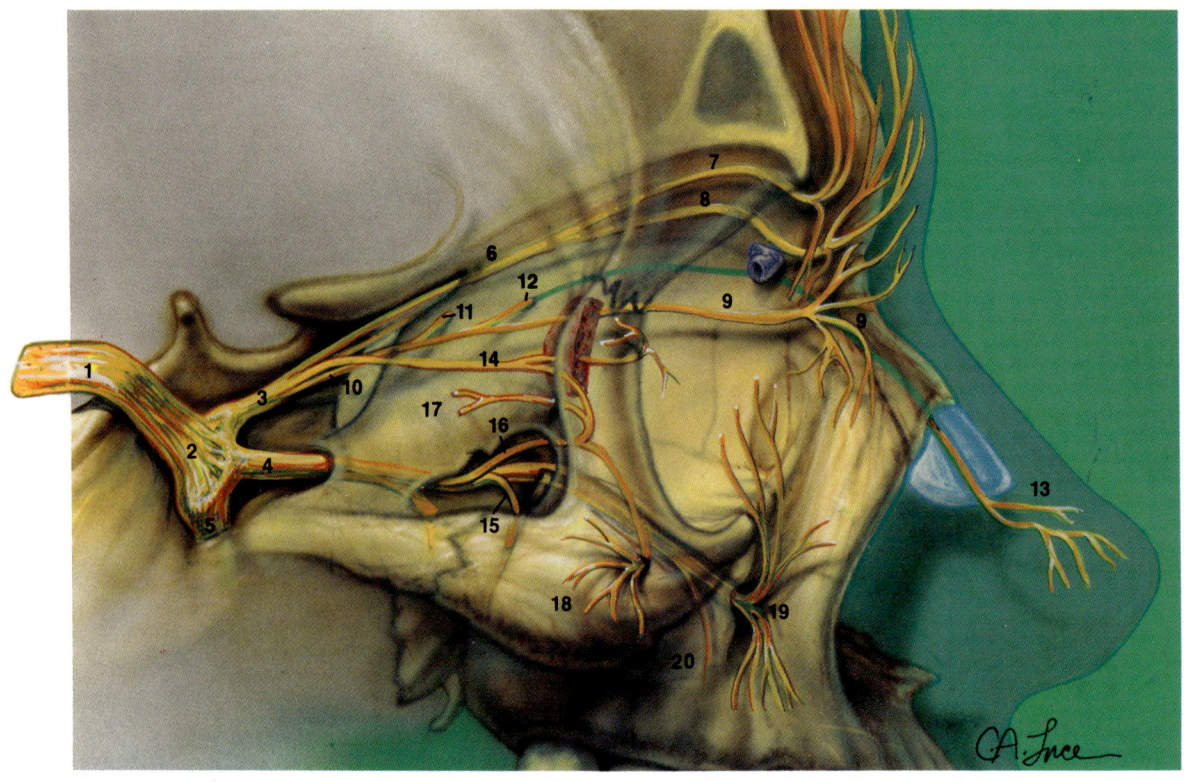

Fig. 1-16. A: Sensory nerves.

(1) cranial nerve V;
(2) trigeminal ganglion;
(3) ophthalmic division of trigeminal nerve V₁;
(4) maxillary division of trigeminal nerve V₂;
(5) mandibular division of trigeminal nerve V₃;
(6) frontal nerve;
(7) supraorbital nerve;
(8) supratrochlear nerve (trochlea noted by *purple*);
(9) infratrochlear nerve;
(10) nasociliary nerve;
(11) posterior ethmoidal nerve;
(12) anterior ethmoidal nerve;
(13) external or dorsal nasal nerve;
(14) lacrimal nerve;
(15) posterior superior alveolar nerve;
(16) zygomatic nerve;
(17) zygomaticotemporal nerve;
(18) zygomaticofacial nerve;
(19) infraorbital nerve; and
(20) anterior superior alveolar nerve.
(21) ciliary ganglion;
(22) nerve to inferior oblique;
(23) sensory root of ciliary ganglion;
(24) long ciliary nerves;
(25) short ciliary nerves.

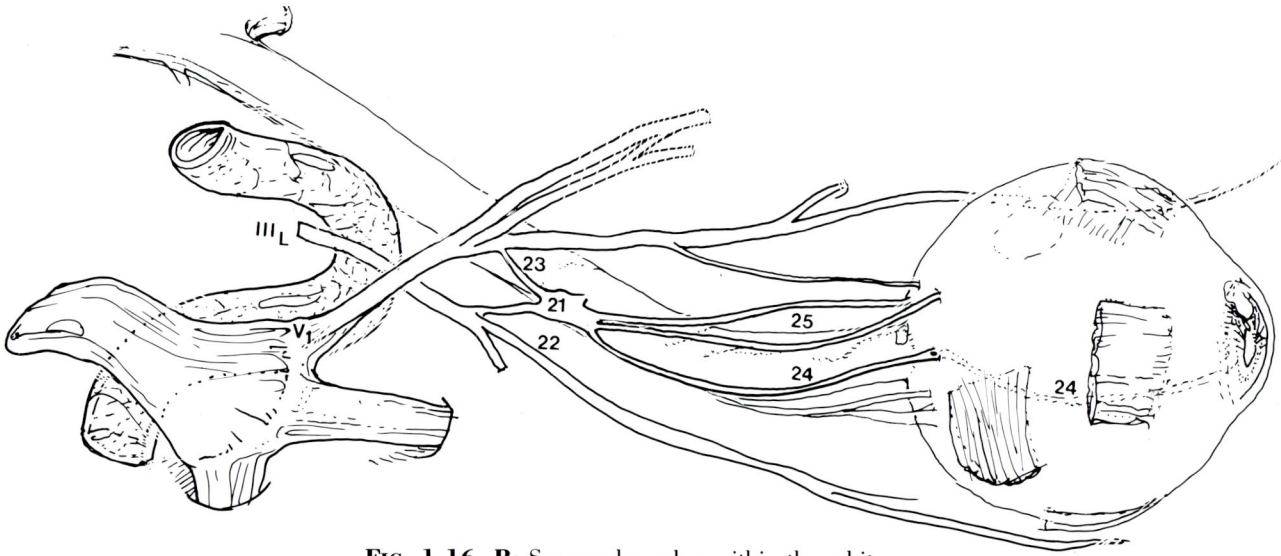

Fig. 1-16. B: Sensory branches within the orbit.

2

Forehead, Temporal Region, and Cheek

Surgical access may be facilitated by dissection through structures around the orbit. By the same token, disease processes within these structures may invade the orbital contents or affect the protection of the eye. Details of the anatomy provide the surgeon with the rationale behind mobilization of these tissues and insights into reconstruction of these areas.

Chapter 2

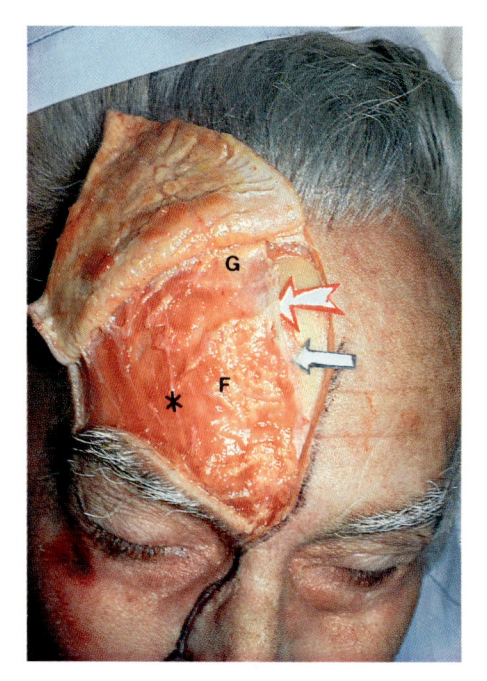

Fig. 2-1. The skin of the forehead is elevated and retracted upward. Note the vertical fibers of the frontalis muscle (F), which insert into the skin and orbicularis oculi at the level of the eyebrow. The frontalis muscle, innervated by a branch of the seventh cranial nerve, originates from the galeal aponeurosis (G). The *red arrow tip* is inserted below the galea. The *black arrow tip* lies beneath the periosteum of the frontal bone. Note the sensory nerve (*), a branch of the supraorbital nerve coursing over the muscle. The frontalis muscle usually does not cross the midline.

Fig. 2-2. Note the paired frontalis muscles (F) with their central muscle-free zone (*). Once again, the supraorbital nerves are noted coursing upward *(small arrows)*. The forceps grasp the anterior portion of the medial canthal tendon. Note the orbicularis oculi fibers (o), some of which originate from this tendon.

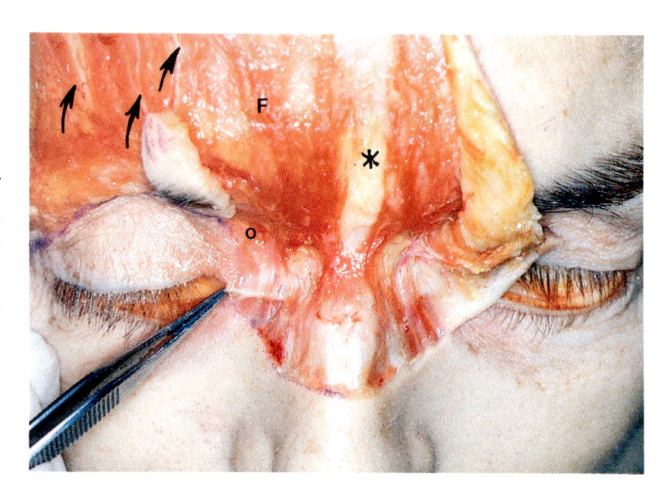

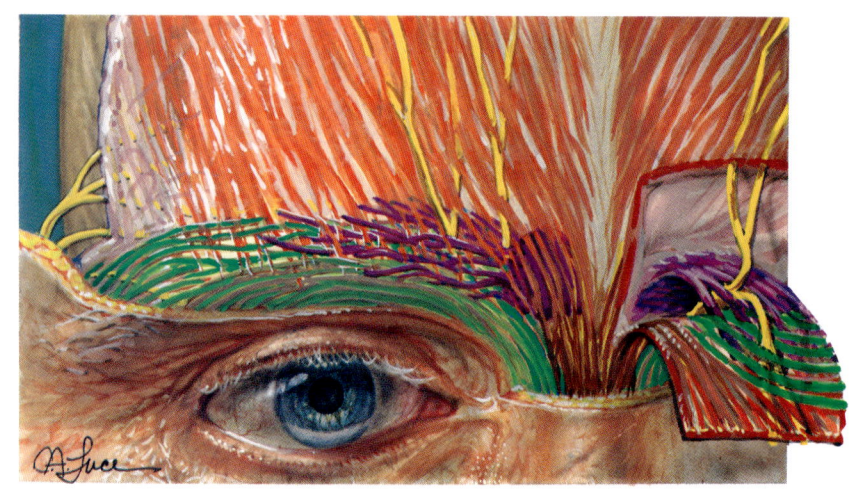

Fig. 2-3. Note the relation of the corrugator muscle *(magenta)* to the surrounding muscles. The procerus muscles *(brown)*, frontalis muscle *(orange)*, and upper orbicularis fibers *(green)* overlie the corrugator.

FOREHEAD, TEMPORAL REGION, AND CHEEK

FIG. 2-4. The frontalis muscle has been excised. Note the edge of the periosteal layer (*) still covering the bone. The corrugator muscle *(red arrow)* arises medially from the frontal bone near the superior medial margin of the orbit beneath the frontalis muscle. It courses laterally and upward to insert into the skin of the medial half of the eyebrow.

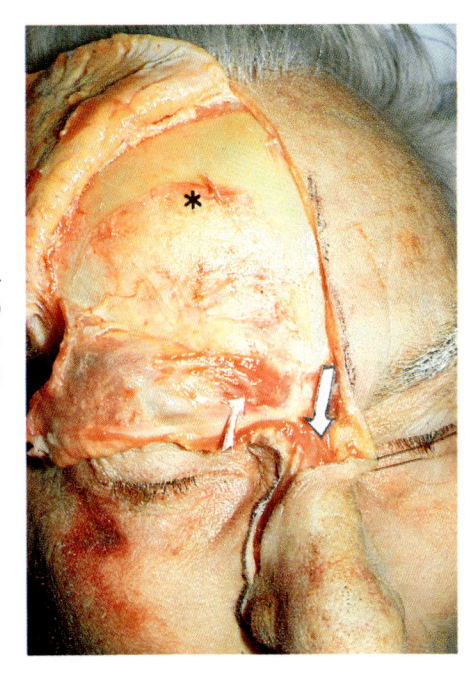

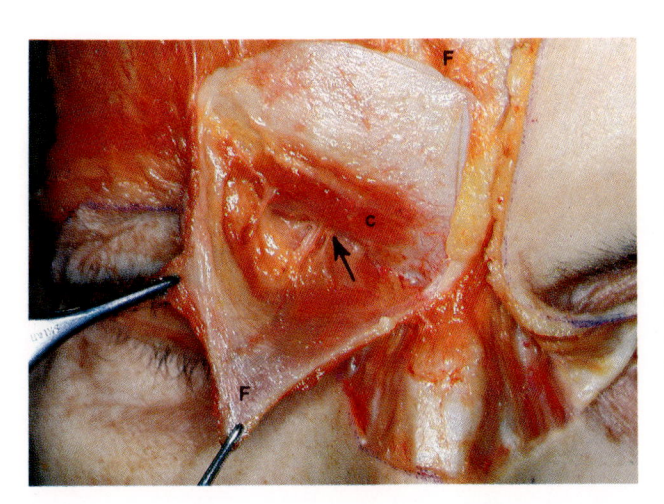

FIG. 2-5. The frontalis muscle (F) is retracted downward and forward. Note that the corrugator muscle (c) and the supraorbital vessels and nerves are passing through the lower portion of the muscle *(arrows)*. Care should be taken to protect these vessels and nerves to prevent considerable bleeding or postoperative numbness after aggressive corrugator resection.

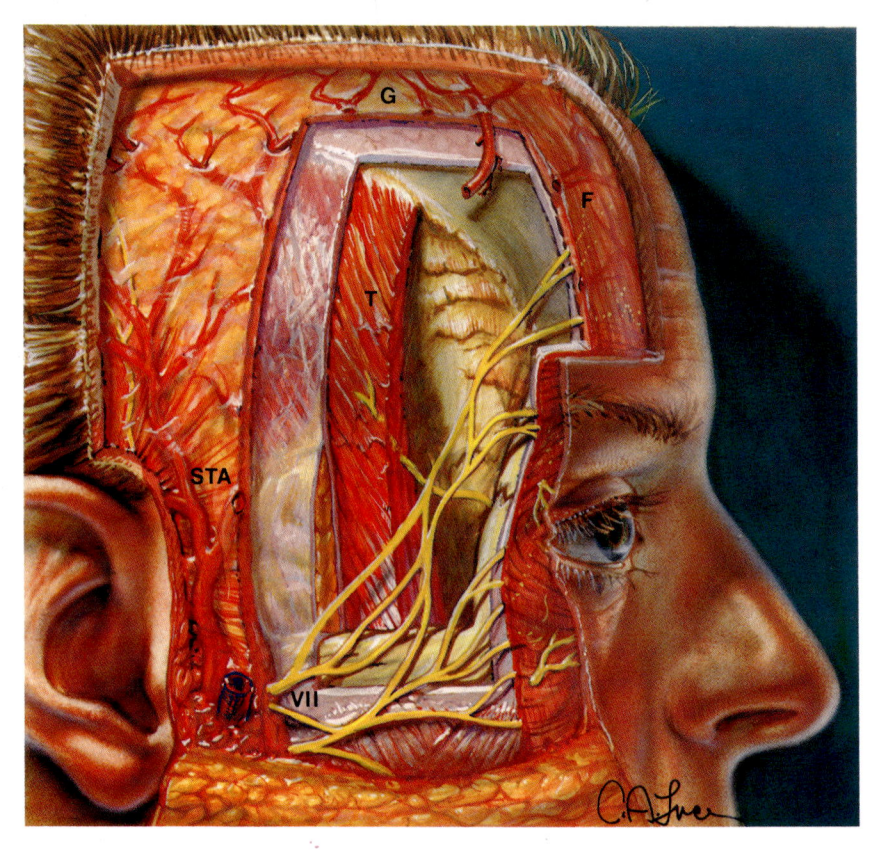

CHAPTER 2

FIG. 2-6. As the frontalis muscle (F) continues posteriorly, it becomes confluent with the galea (G). The superficial temporal vessels (STA) lie within the superficial temporal fascia, which is continuous with the galea. More cephalad, the vessels course just over the galea. Below this superficial fascia, note the thicker glistening deeper layer of superficial temporal fascia (often termed temporalis fascia) that lies adherent to the temporalis muscle (T). As this deeper fascia continues inferiorly, it splits to envelop first fat and then the zygomatic arch. The fascia is fused with the periosteum of the zygoma. The frontal or temporal branch of the facial nerve (VII) lies on the periosteum of the proximal one-third of the zygomatic arch. This is usually 2.5 cm from the anterior border external auditory meatus, but may vary between 0.8 and 3.5 cm from this point. The course of the nerve is oblique, passing approximately 1.5 cm lateral to the lateral brow to enter the frontalis muscle on its undersurface not greater than 2 cm above the eyebrow. The branch innervates the muscles of the brow: frontalis, corrugator, procerus, and occasionally a portion of the orbicularis oculi. All muscles are innervated from their posterior surfaces.

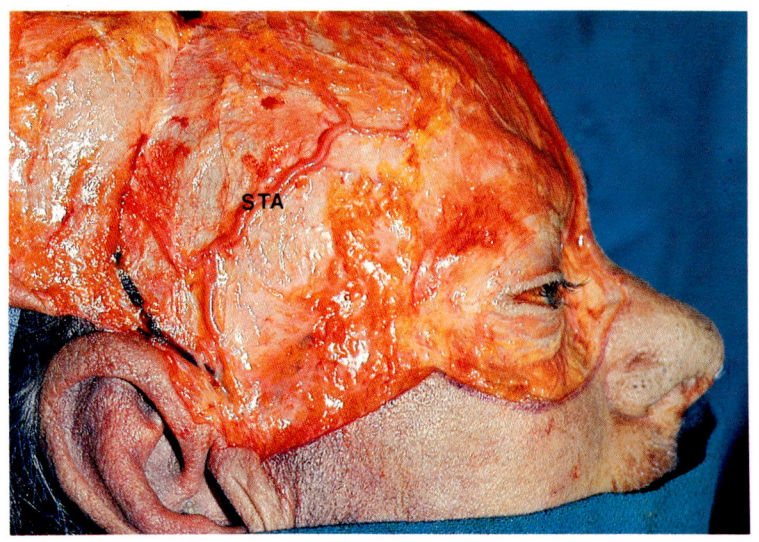

FIG. 2-7. Note the superficial temporal artery (STA), which lies within the superficial temporal fascia. This fascia is continuous superiorly with the galea.

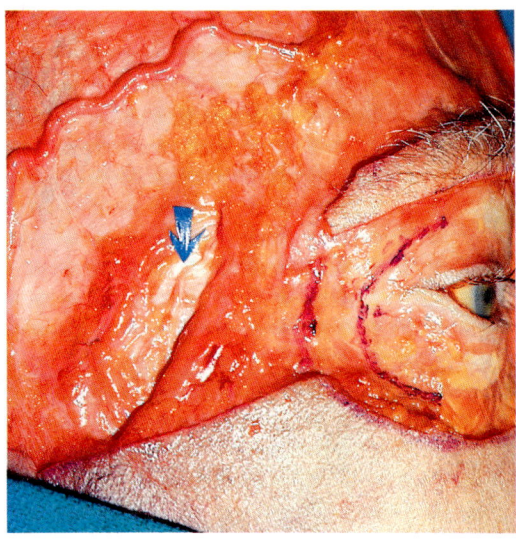

FIG. 2-8. Purple dye outlines the frontal process of the zygoma. An incision through the superficial fascia reveals the frontal branch of the facial nerve *(arrow)* approximately 1.5 cm lateral to the lateral brow. It is evident from the dissection that this nerve lies deep to the fascia.

FOREHEAD, TEMPORAL REGION, AND CHEEK

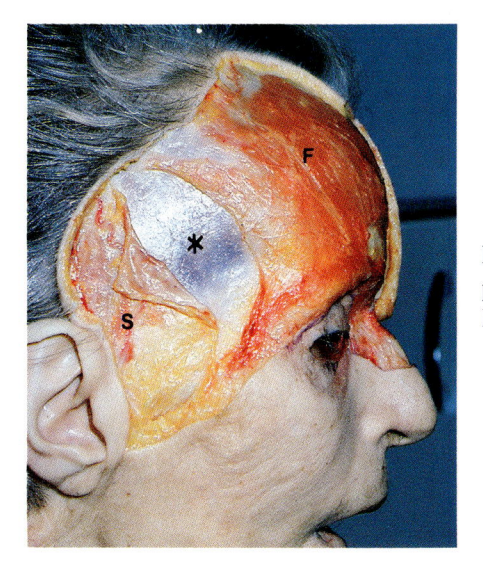

FIG. 2-9. An incision is made between the frontalis muscle (F) and the superficial temporal fascial layer containing the superficial temporal vessels (S). Note the glistening temporalis fascia which overlies the muscle (*).

FIG. 2-10. The superficial temporal fascia is retracted posteriorly. Note the cut edge of frontalis muscle (F). The *small arrows* outline the superior temporal line, where the temporalis fascia begins. The temporalis muscle lies below this line. The *dotted line* denotes the point at which the temporalis fascia splits prior to enveloping the zygomatic arch (Z).

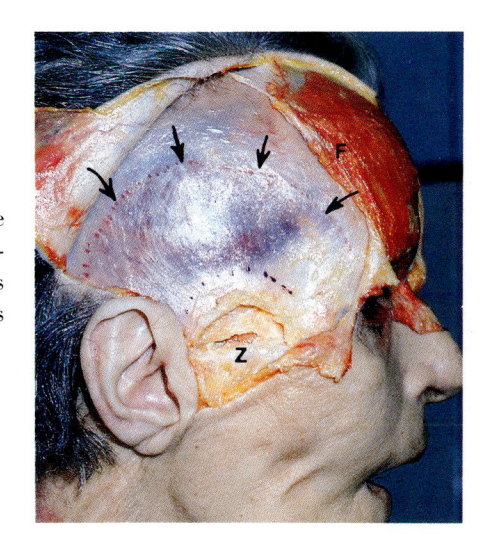

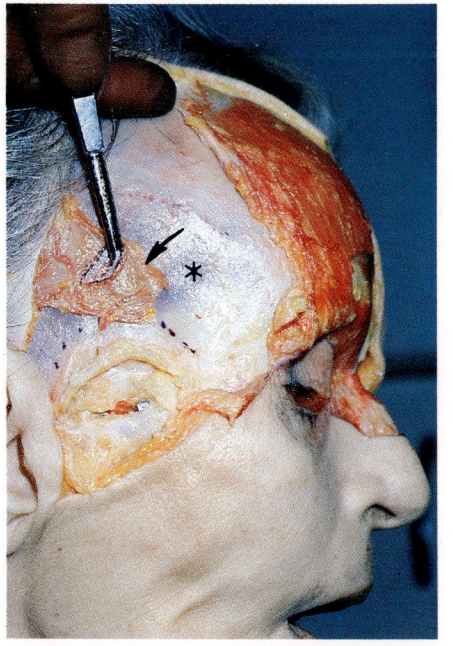

FIG. 2-11. It is important to understand the relationship of the superficial and deep layers of the temporal fascia in relation to the zygomatic arch when reducing fractures. In order to elevate a fractured zygomatic bone or its arch, the elevator must be placed beneath both layers above the point of fusion at which deeper layer splits (dotted). This allows access to the medial aspect of the bone. In this dissection, a small remnant of superficial temporal fascia *(arrow)* has been preserved overlying the deeper temporalis fascia (*). The elevator pierces both layers to lie on the surface of the temporalis muscle. Passage inferiorly provides access to the medial zygoma (Gillies maneuver).

Chapter 2

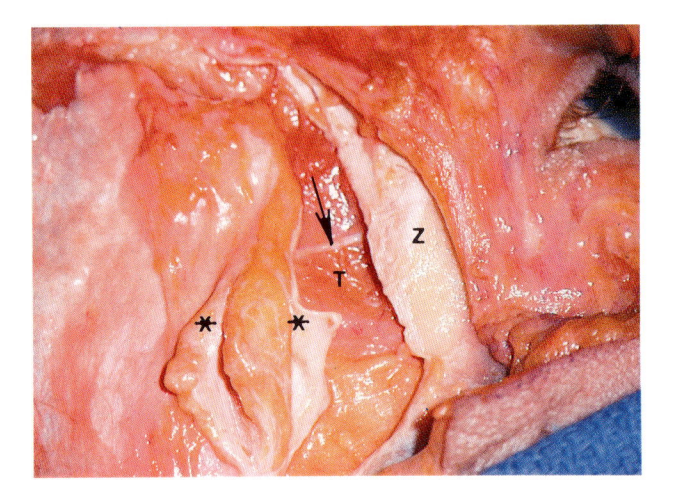

Fig. 2-12. Note the frontal process of the zygoma (Z). The cut edge of temporalis fascia is retracted to expose the temporalis muscle (T) below. Note the split temporalis fascia (*) and enclosed fat pad. Another pad of fat can be found on the surface of the muscle. The zygomaticotemporal nerve *(arrow)* crosses the temporalis muscle to later supply sensation to the skin of the temporal region.

Fig. 2-13. The superficial temporal fascia has been incised and reflected anteriorly and inferiorly with the periosteum over the lateral orbital rim and zygoma (Z). The retractor exposes the tendinous origin of the masseter muscle (M). Note a zygomaticofacial nerve *(arrow)* as it exits from its foramen. This nerve supplies sensation to tissues over the zygoma and the lateral lower lid.

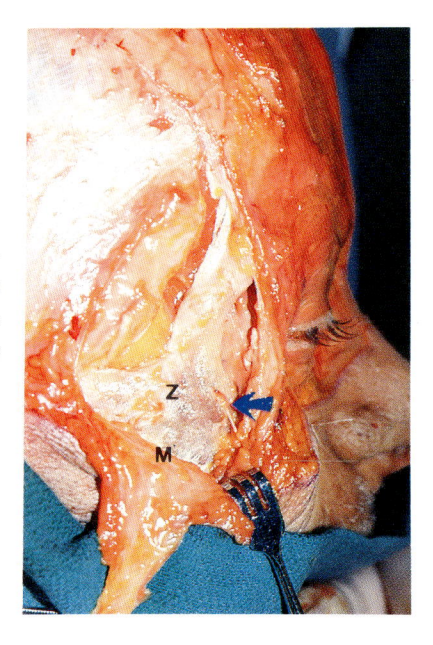

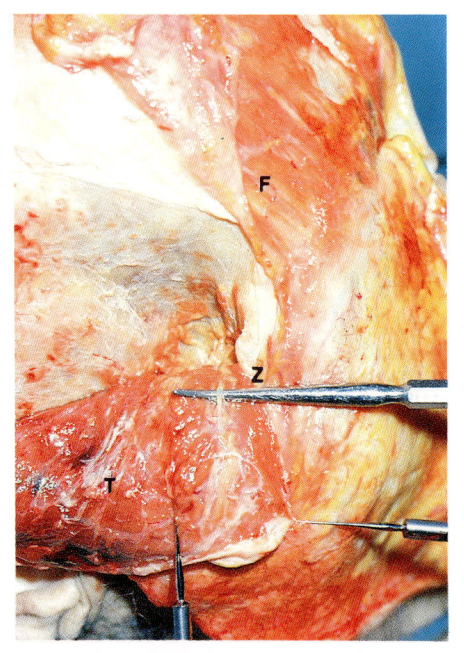

Fig. 2-14. The temporalis muscle (T) is elevated and retracted to expose the temporal fossa. The probe is passed under the anterior deep temporal nerve, which innervates the temporalis muscle. From its medial surface, the deep temporal vessels enter the muscle in a similar location. Note the zygomatic bone (Z) and frontalis muscle (F).

FOREHEAD, TEMPORAL REGION, AND CHEEK

FIG. 2-15. Much of the skin and fat of the cheek and nose has been excised. Note the orbicularis oculi muscle (o.o.) with an oblique extension onto the cheek. This muscle medially overlaps the levator labii superioris (L) and the levator of the ala of the nose (La).

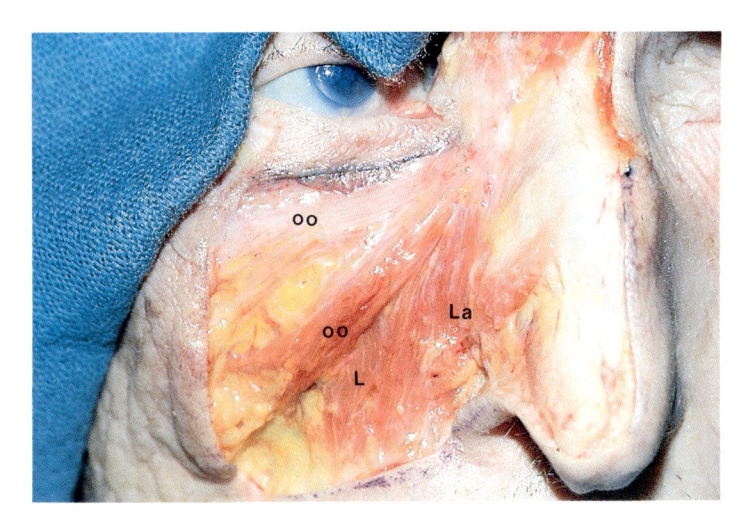

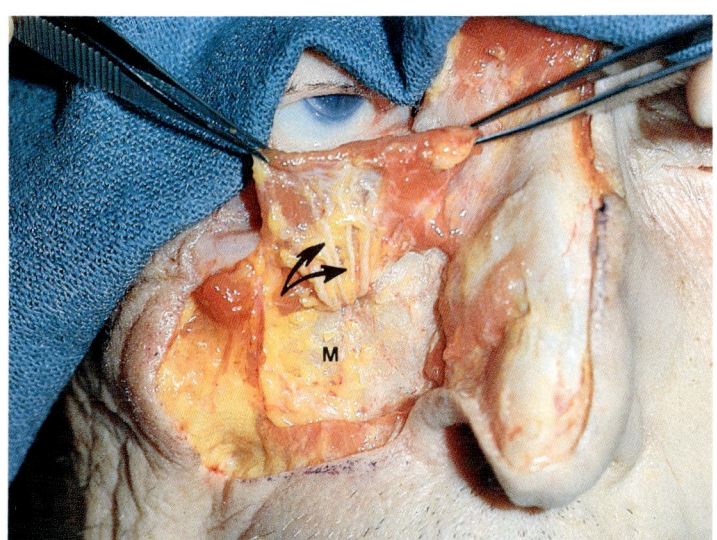

FIG. 2-16. The elevator muscles are incised and lifted with forceps to expose the underlying anterior maxilla (M). Note the infraorbital nerve branches *(arrow)* adherent to the underside of the levator muscle complex.

FIG. 2-17. Cheek muscle (diagrammatic): (1) orbicularis oculi *(orange)*; (2) nasalis transversus *(yellow)*; (3) levator of nasal ala *(green)*; (4) levator labii superioris *(pink)*; (5) levator anguli oris *(blue)*; (6) zygomaticus minor *(dark green)*; and (7) zygomaticus major *(red)*.

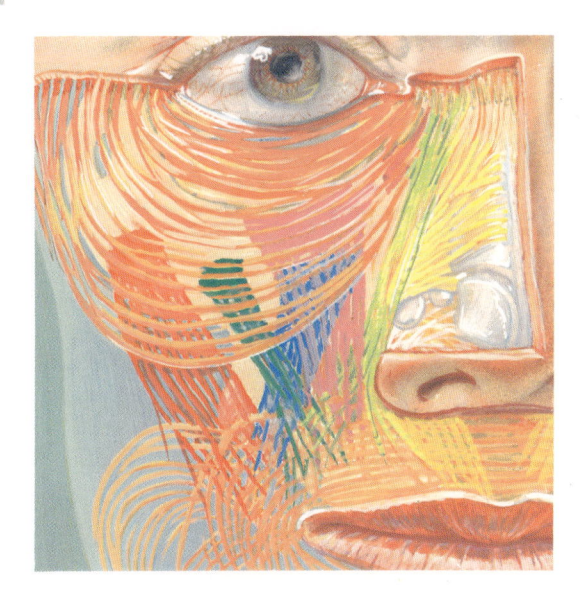

19

3
The Eyelids

The eyelids contain specialized structures that protect the eyes from excessive light, exposure to extremes of the elements, and airborne debris. During blinking, they distribute a protective and optically important tear film over the cornea.

Chapter 3

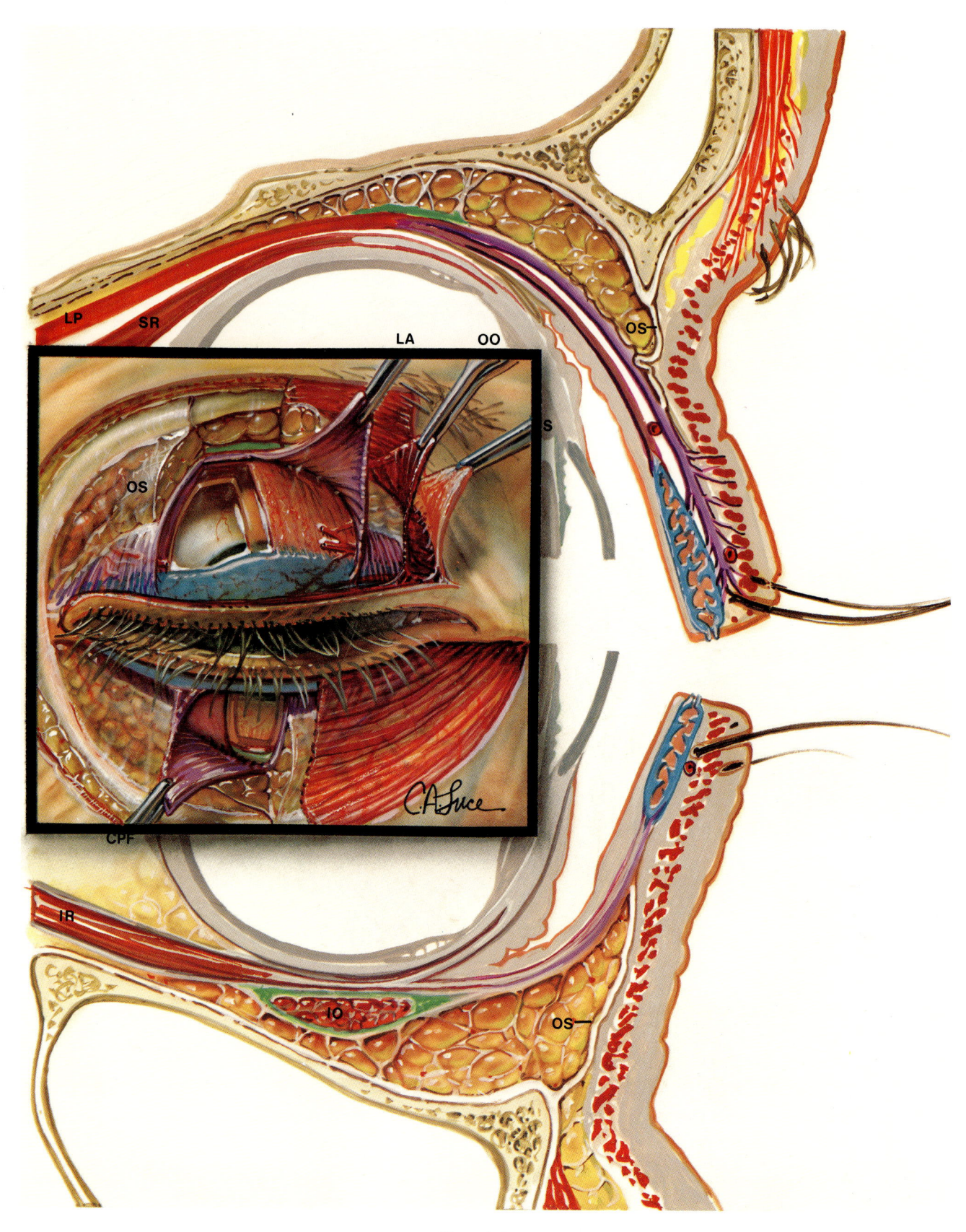

Fig. 3-1.

THE EYELIDS

FIG. 3-1. This illustration depicts those structures of the upper and lower eyelids and orbit that are considered anatomically and functionally analogous. The structures are color coded and are presented in a cross-sectional as well as anterior-layered dissection format: eyelid skin and subcutaneous tissue *(light orange and grey, respectively)*; orbicularis oculi muscle *(red)*; orbital septum (OS) *(white)*; tarsi *(blue)*; orbital fat *(yellow)*; upper eyelid levator aponeurosis and lower eyelid aponeurosis (extension of capsulopalpebral fascia to inferior border of tarsus) *(purple)*; upper eyelid, Muller's muscle and lower eyelid, inferior tarsal (Horner's muscle) *(salmon)*; upper eyelid, Whitnall's ligament (superior transverse ligament) and lower eyelid, Lockwood's ligament (inferior transverse suspensory ligament) *(green)*. Other structures shown: inferior oblique muscle (IO); superior rectus muscle (SR); inferior rectus muscle (IR); and levator palpebrae muscle (LP).

FIG. 3-2. For convenience, the upper eyelid may be divided into anterior and posterior segments or lamellae. The anterior lamella consists of the skin and orbicularis muscle and its associated fascial and vascular structures. Note the marginal artery *(lower arrow)* approximately 3 to 3.5 mm above the lid margin. The posterior lamella consists of the levator aponeurosis (L), tarsus *(blue)*, Muller's muscle (M), and conjunctival lining (c). At a variable height above the superior edge of the tarsus, the orbital septum (o.s.) forms the anterior border of the preaponeurotic fat space. The peripheral arterial arcade *(upper arrow)* is situated at the level of the superior edge of the tarsus posterior to the levator aponeurosis within the so-called pretarsal space.

The levator muscle (the primary elevator of the upper lid) usually becomes aponeurotic at the equator of the globe in the superior orbit. The aponeurosis courses anteriorly to insert onto the lower two-thirds of the anterior tarsal plate. The levator muscle provides origin to Muller's muscle (M), the non-striated, sympathetically-innervated elevator of the upper lid, which inserts into the superior edge of the tarsus. The superior transverse ligament of Whitnall (W) is noted as a fascial condensation along the upper aspect of the levator muscle. This ligament attaches to the trochlear fascia medially and the fascia of the orbital lobe of the lacrimal gland laterally.

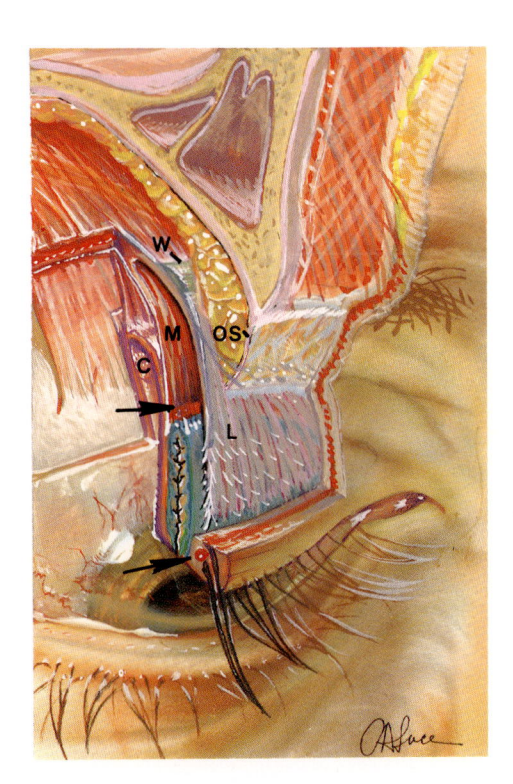

Chapter 3

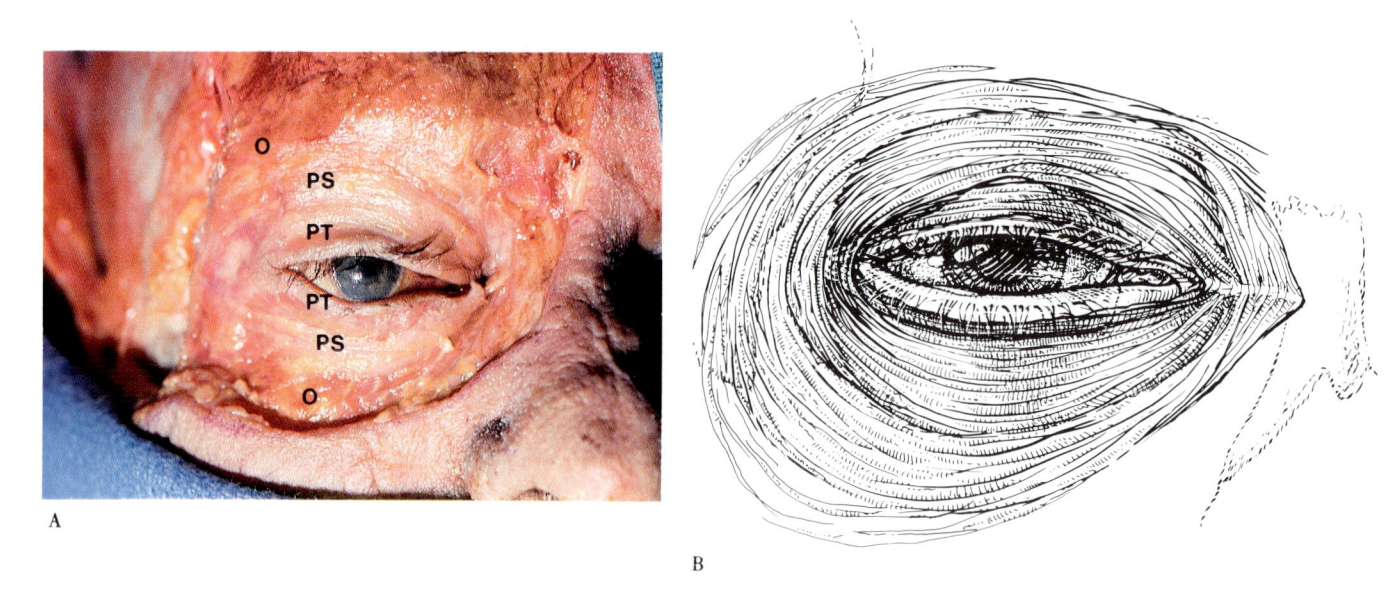

Fig. 3-3. A & B: The periorbital skin has been removed, exposing orbicularis oculi muscle that is innervated by the seventh cranial nerve. This muscle acts as an antagonist to the levator palpebrae superioris muscle innervated by the third cranial nerve.

The orbicularis oculi muscle is divided into palpebral and orbital portions. The palpebral portion is further subdivided into pretarsal (PT) and preseptal (PS) portions.

The orbital portion (o) of the orbicularis oculi arises medially from the superomedial orbital margin, the maxillary process of the frontal bone, the medial canthal tendon, the frontal process of the maxilla, and the inferomedial orbital margin. The peripheral fibers sweep across the eyelid over the orbital margin in a series of concentric loops, the more central ones forming almost complete rings. In the upper lid, the orbital portion spreads upward onto the forehead, covers the corrugator supercilii muscle, and continues laterally over the anterior temporalis fascia. In the lower lid, the orbital portion covers the origins of the elevator muscles of the upper lip and nasal ala and continues temporally to cover part of the origin of the masseter muscle. Occasionally, the lower orbital portion may actually continue downward into the cheek. The preseptal portion diverges from its origin on the medial canthal tendon and lacrimal diaphragm and passes across the lid as a series of half ellipses to meet at the lateral canthal raphe. The muscle bundles are not interrupted and do not interdigitate at the raphe. The pretarsal muscles form a common lateral canthal tendon approximately 7 mm from the lateral orbital tubercle where it inserts. The insertion is 7 to 10 mm from the zygomaticofrontal suture. Medially, the orbicularis oculi unites to join the medial canthal tendon, which inserts on the medial orbital margin and nasal bones.

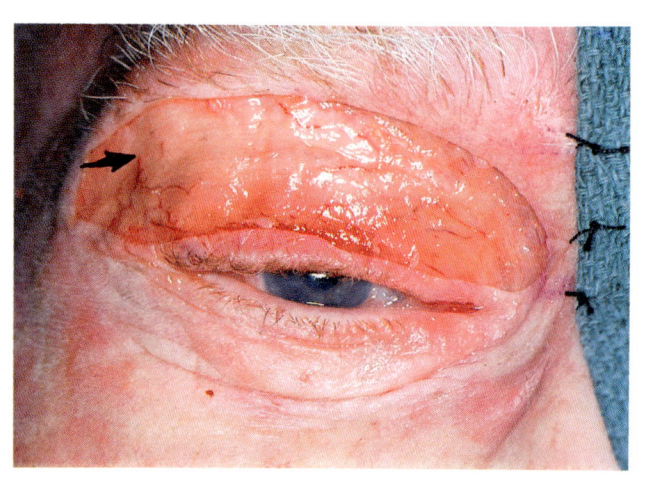

Fig. 3-4. A rich anastomotic arterial network supplies the upper lid. The terminal branches of the lacrimal artery *(arrow)* pass around or through the lacrimal gland to become upper lateral palpebral branches. These anastomose with the medial palpebral branches, easily seen in this specimen. More deeply, these vessels unite, forming the marginal and peripheral arterial arcades of the lid. The marginal arterial arcade is located 3 to 3.5 mm superior to the lid margin, deep to the orbicularis muscle. The peripheral arterial arcade courses beneath the levator aponeurosis at the superior border of the tarsal plate. The venous drainage generally parallels the arterial supply.

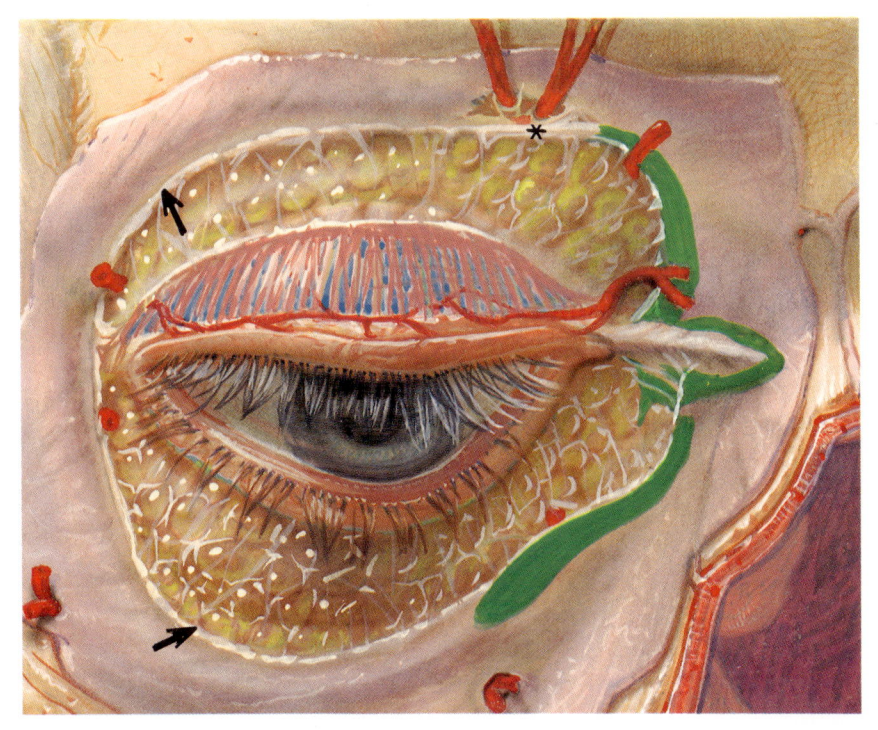

THE EYELIDS

FIG. 3-5. The *green* outline denotes the medial origins of the orbicularis oculi muscle. The orbital septum is a fascial membrane that separates the eyelid structures from the deeper orbital structures. It is a barrier that helps prevent the spread of hemorrhage, infection, inflammation, and other disease processes.

The orbital septum attaches to the orbital margin at a thickening called the arcus marginalis *(arrows)*. The arcus marginalis is also the point of confluence for the facial bone periosteum and the periorbita. The orbital septum is usually thicker laterally in both lids. Although the attachment follows the orbital margin for the most part, some key anatomic points must be made: First, laterally, the orbital septum lies in front of the lateral canthal tendon (although this is disputed). Second, superomedially, the arcus marginalis usually forms the inferior part of the supraorbital groove (*). Therefore the supraorbital neurovascular structures frequently exit from a groove or notch closed by the arcus marginalis. Third, medially, the orbital septum passes in front of the superior oblique trochlear pulley and then runs backward behind the deep heads of the orbicularis oculi onto the posterior lacrimal crest. Fourth, the orbital septum follows the rim along the inferior portion of the anterior lacrimal crest and inferior orbital rim. Finally, in the lateral half of the orbital rim, the orbital septum actually originates a few millimeters inferior to the temporal orbital margin, forming a potential space on the facial aspect of the zygoma (the recess of Eisler, lower arrow).

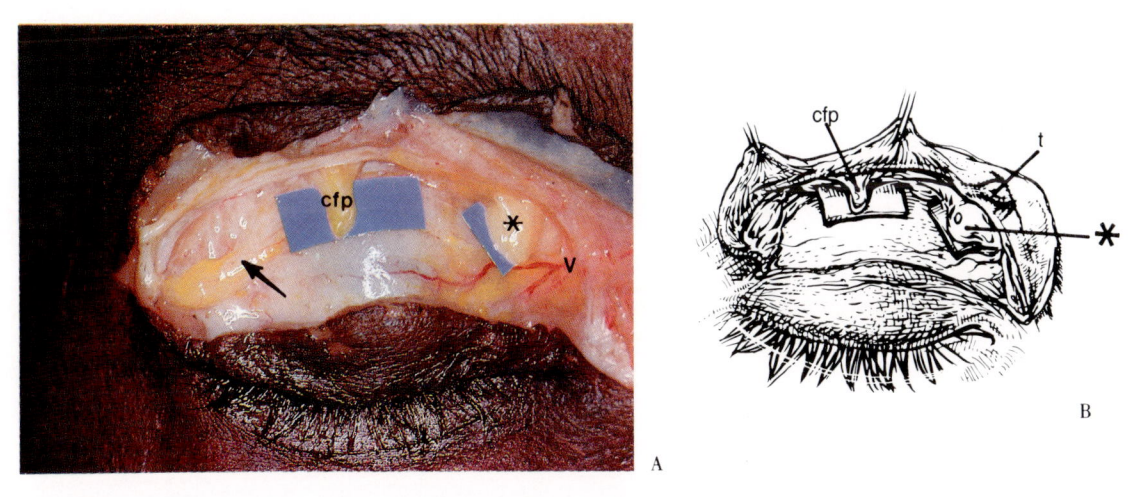

FIG. 3-6. A: The medial palpebral arterial vessels (v) can be seen separating into marginal and peripheral components. A superficial medial fat pad (*) and a central fat pad (cfp) are not particularly large; however, some of the central fat pad extends to the lateral upper lid *(arrow)*. The orbital portion of the lacrimal gland may be seen extending superior to this lateral fat pad. **B:** The medial or nasal fat compartment may be found inferior to the trochlea (t). After passage through the trochlea, the superior oblique tendon is directed posterolaterally to insert on the globe. An intricate sheath surrounds the tendon to provide an efficient low-friction gliding path. Injury to the trochlea or its associated structures may result in extraocular muscle imbalance.

Chapter 3

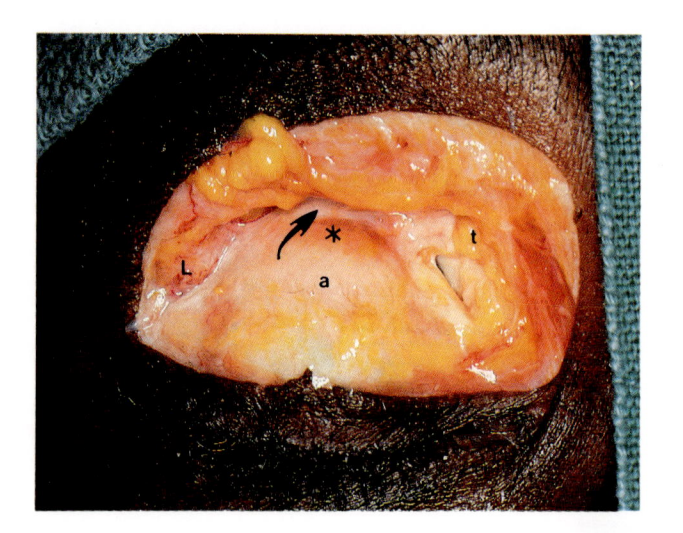

Fig. 3-7. In this dissection, the orbital septum and preaponeurotic fat have been elevated to expose Whitnall's ligament *(arrow)* as a fascial condensation or ligamentous band stretching across the orbit superior to the levator muscle (*) and its aponeurosis (LA). Medially, the fibers connect to the trochlea (t), but some fibers actually pass to bone and bridge the supraorbital notch. Laterally, Whitnall's ligament joins the lacrimal gland stroma (L) and fascia.

Fig. 3-8. A & B: The aponeurotic expansion of the levator palpebrae superioris usually commences a few millimeters beyond the equator of the globe. This aponeurosis fans out, molding itself on the globe. It inserts onto the anterior surface of the tarsus as well as into the fascia between the bundles of orbicularis oculi. The levator aponeurosis has been detached from the anterior tarsus and reflected upward. Laterally and medially, the aponeurosis possesses "horns" or cornua. The lateral horn passes between the orbital and palpebral portions of the lacrimal gland (L). Medially, the horn attaches to the medial orbital wall. In this view, the aponeurosis (LA) is rolled up with the forceps to expose Muller's muscle (M) inserting onto the superior edge of the tarsus (T).

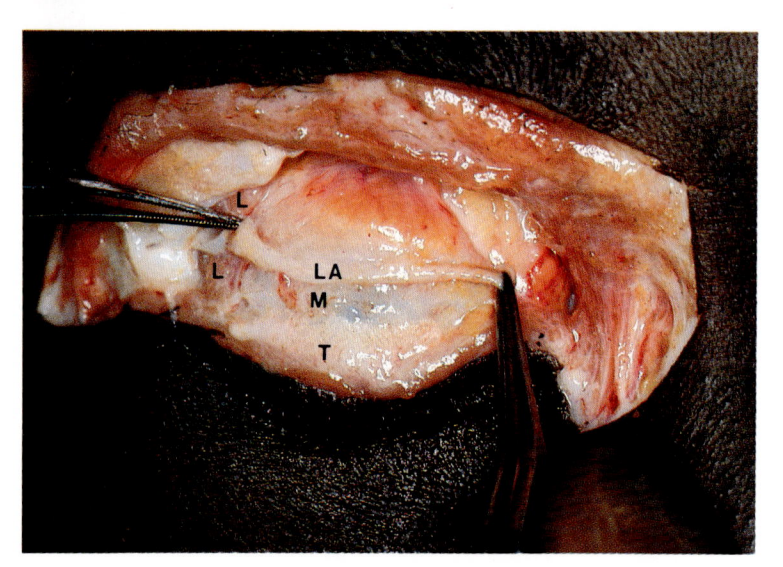

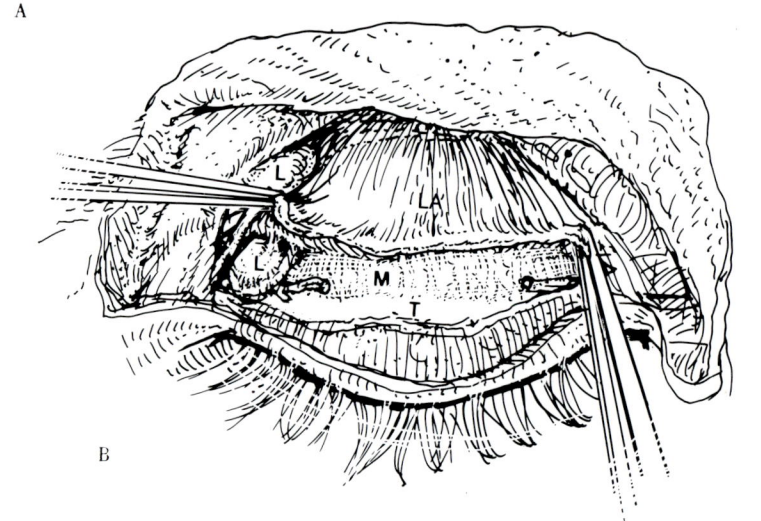

26

THE EYELIDS

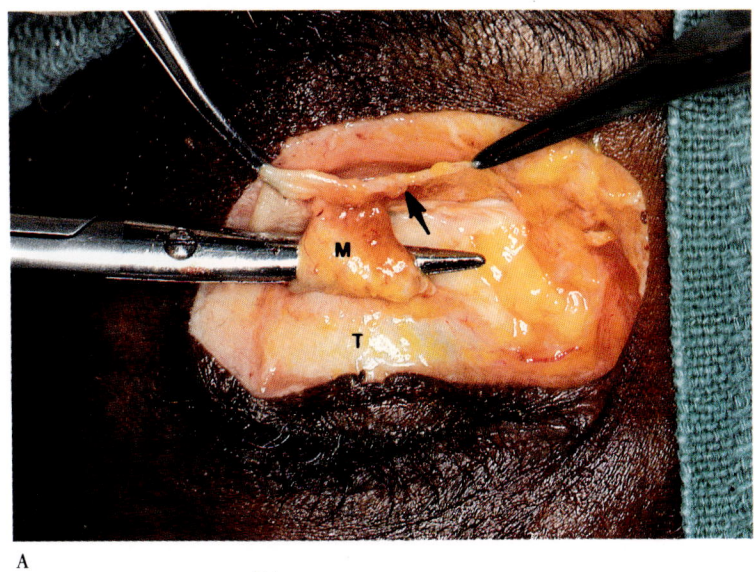

FIG. 3-9. A & B: Muller's muscle (M) is noted originating from the underside of the muscular portion of the levator *(arrow)*. This nonstriated muscle inserts into the superior border of the tarsal plate (T).

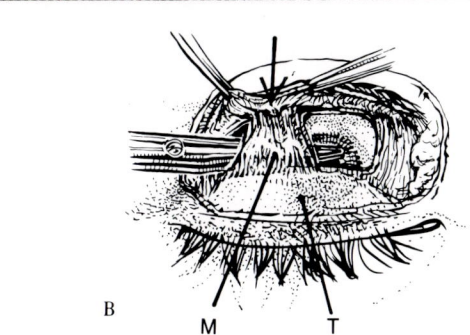

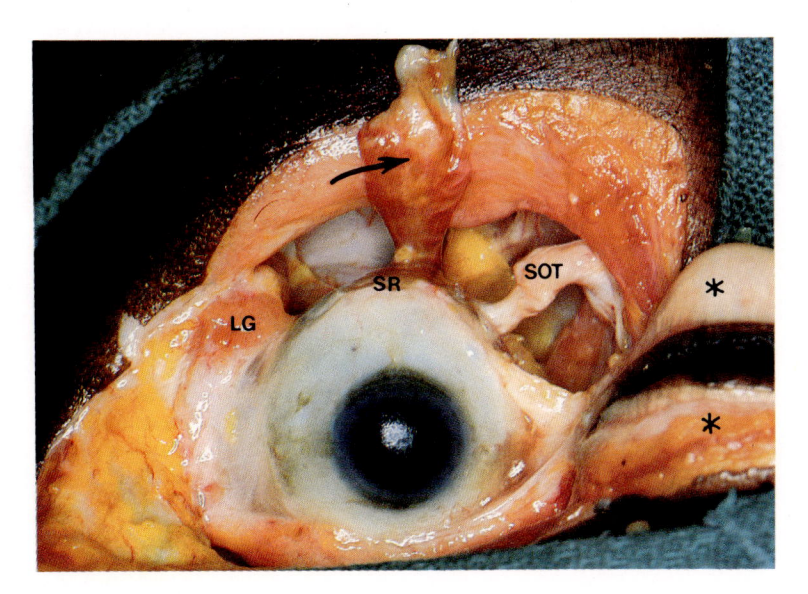

FIG. 3-10. The levator aponeurosis and Muller's muscle *(arrow)* are detached from the upper lid and reflected superiorly. The upper and lower eyelids (*) have been detached from the lateral orbital tubercle and are reflected medially. The superior rectus muscle (SR), the superior oblique tendon (SOT), and the orbital lobe of the lacrimal gland (LG) can now be seen. The tendon of the superior oblique muscle separates the central fat from the nasal fat compartment.

27

CHAPTER 3

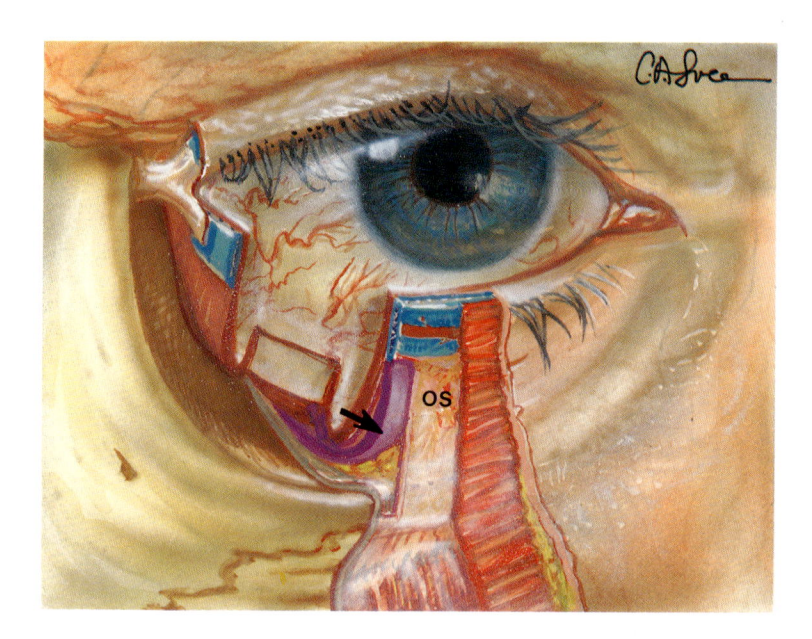

FIG. 3-11. The anterior lamella of the lower lid consists of skin and underlying muscle. Note the cut edge of the orbital septum (OS), which meets at the junction of periosteum and periorbita, the arcus marginalis. The *arrow* denotes the capsulopalpebral fascia, an extension of the inferior rectus muscle that acts to lower the eyelid in unison with the globe during downward gaze. A well-developed nonstriated muscle is usually not seen in the lower lid complex.

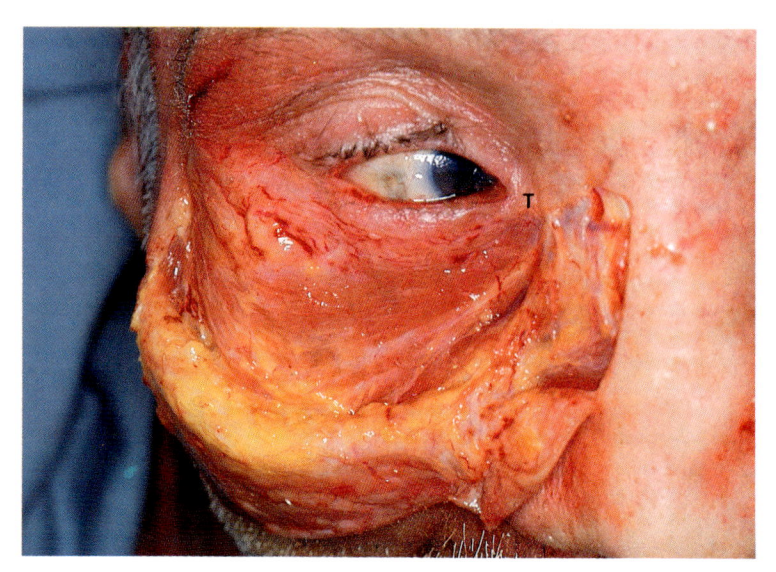

FIG. 3-12. The skin of the lower eyelid is retracted inferiorly, exposing the orbicularis oculi muscle. Note the horizontal orientation of the blood supply in the upper portion of the muscle. These represent branches of the inferior medial and lateral palpebral branches derived from the infratrochlear and lacrimal arteries, respectively. The arterial supply courses in a submuscular plane and receives anastomosing twigs from the angular infraorbital, transverse facial, and zygomaticofacial vessels.

Note that the orbicularis oculi muscle originates from the medial canthal tendon (T) and from the lower orbital margin medial to the infraorbital foramen. The orbicularis fibers sweep temporally, often covering the origins of the elevators of the upper lip and nasal ala. They extend across the cheek to overlie the anterior part of temporalis fascia. The motor nerve supply enters the muscle laterally via the zygomatic branches of the facial nerve. Venous drainage generally follows the course of the arterial supply. Lymphatic drainage from the lateral side is into the preauricular and parotid nodes. The medial side drains into the submandibular regional nodes.

THE EYELIDS

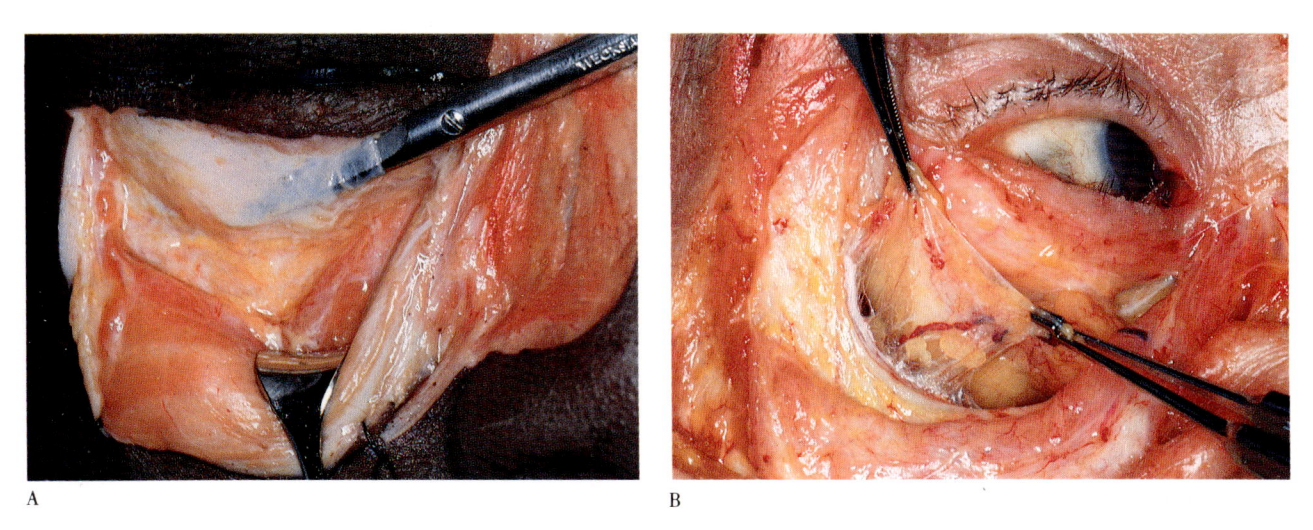

FIG. 3-13. The thickness of the orbital septum varies from lid to lid, from person to person, and from location to location in the same lid. **A:** In this dissection of the orbit of a 25-year-old male, a substantial orbital septum is observed overlying the scissor blades. The most medial portion of the septum is somewhat thinner. **B:** The orbital septum of this 85-year-old specimen is extremely thin.

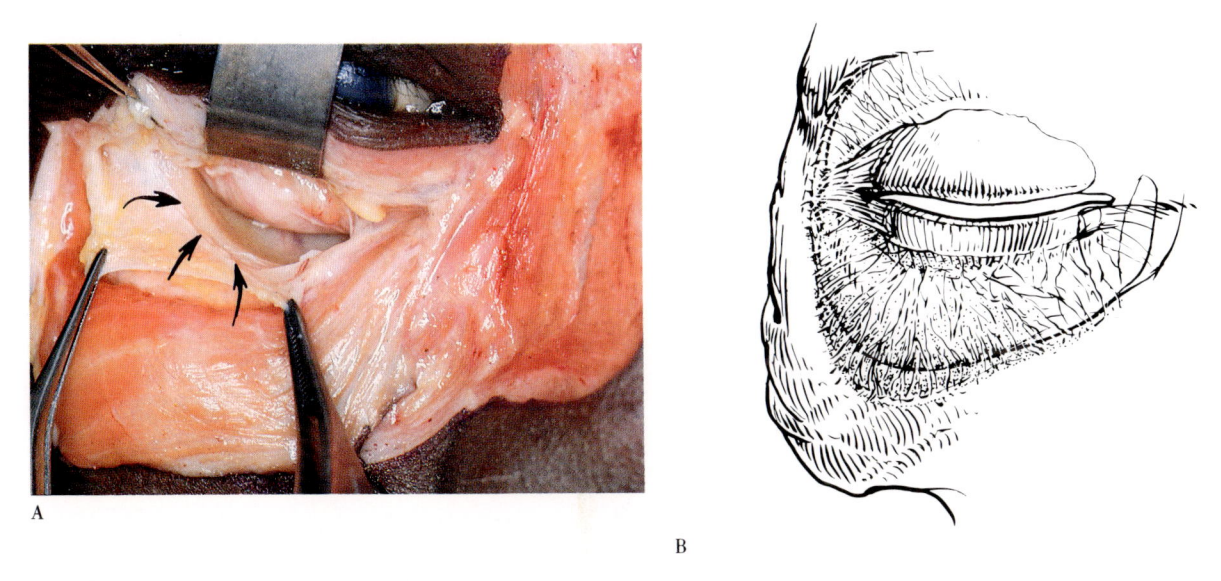

FIG. 3-14. **A:** The forceps retract the orbital septum forward, exposing the arcus marginalis on the inferolateral orbital rim. The septum originates directly from the orbital margin medially; however, the origin drifts downward onto the face of the maxilla as it progresses laterally *(arrows)*. Thus, incisions to expose fractures at the rim and to explore the orbital floor should drop slightly as one incises laterally. The malleable retractor elevates the orbital contents to expose the orbital floor. **B.** Orbital septum insertion inferiorly (diagrammatic).

29

Chapter 3

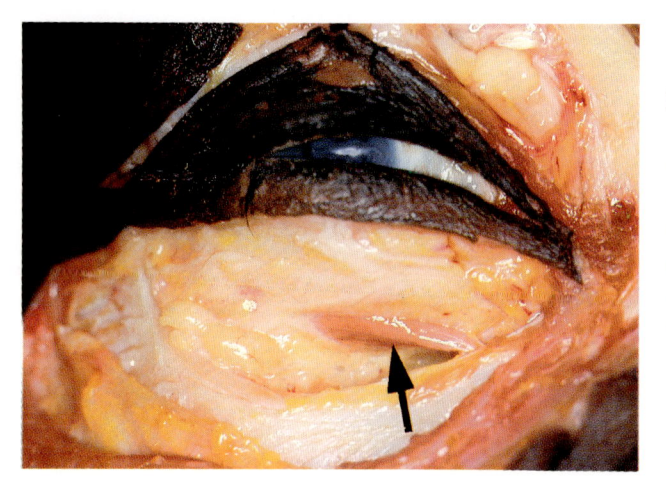

Fig. 3-15. The inferior oblique muscle *(arrow)* arises from a small depression or roughness on the orbital plate of the maxilla just behind the margin and slightly lateral to the bony nasolacrimal canal. The only extrinsic muscle to originate from the front of the orbit then courses posterolaterally on a path similar to that of the superior oblique tendon. The upper aspect of the muscle is first in contact with fat. It then courses inferior to the inferior rectus prior to spreading out and inserting onto the posterior temporal aspect of the globe.

Fig. 3-16. The inferior oblique muscle (supplied by the inferior division of the oculomotor nerve) is noted (*). The muscle penetrates the bulbar fascia just as it nears the inferior rectus. The lower portion of this fascia is condensed to form a hammock-type ligament that supports the globe. The anterior portion of this suspensory ligament of Lockwood can be appreciated *(arrows)*. This structure may prevent ocular descent after partial maxillectomy. Lockwood's ligament attaches laterally and forms part of the lateral retinaculum (see Chapter 6). The medial attachment is in the region of the medial orbital wall.

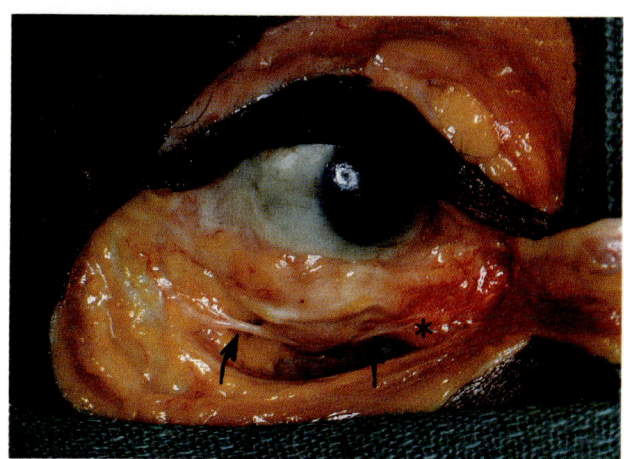

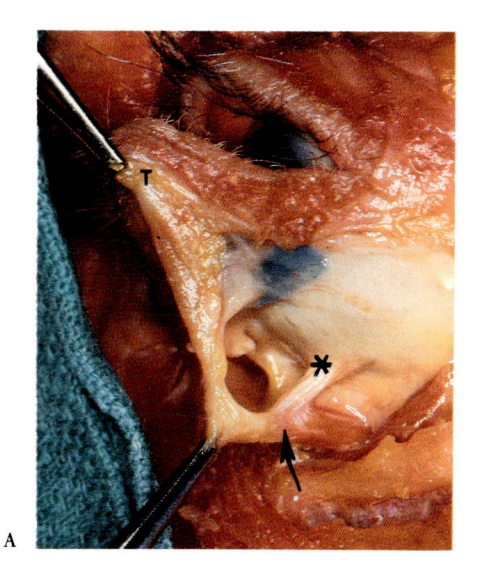

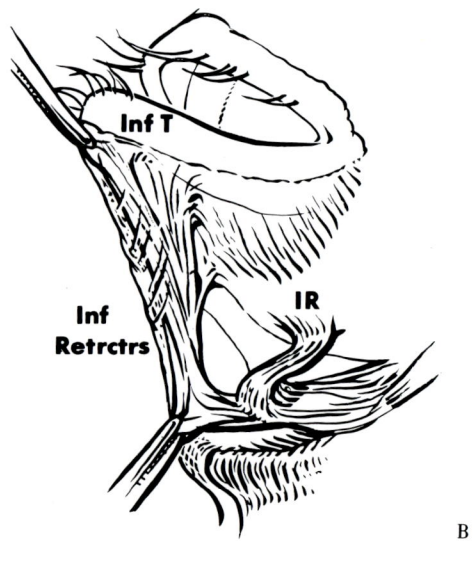

Fig. 3-17. A & B: A piece of blue rubber has been placed in the inferior cul-de-sac. The orbital septum has been completely removed. The lower forceps grasp the capsulopalpebral head just as it comes off the inferior rectus muscle *(arrow)*. This capsulopalpebral fascia is known as the lower lid retractor system and can be seen inserting onto the lower border of the tarsus (T) and conjunctival fornix. The tendinous insertion of the inferior rectus onto the globe can be seen (*). Also arising from this capsulopalpebral fascia (or lower lid retractor) is the nonstriated inferior palpebral muscle, the counterpart to Muller's muscle in the upper lids.

THE EYELIDS

FIG. 3-18. The upper and lower eyelids have been detached from the lateral orbital tubercle and reflected medially. The orbital fat has been removed, exposing the inferior orbit.

The inferior oblique muscle has been said to separate the medial lower lid compartment from the lateral region. The infraorbital nerve is visible below the thin orbital floor *(arrow)*.

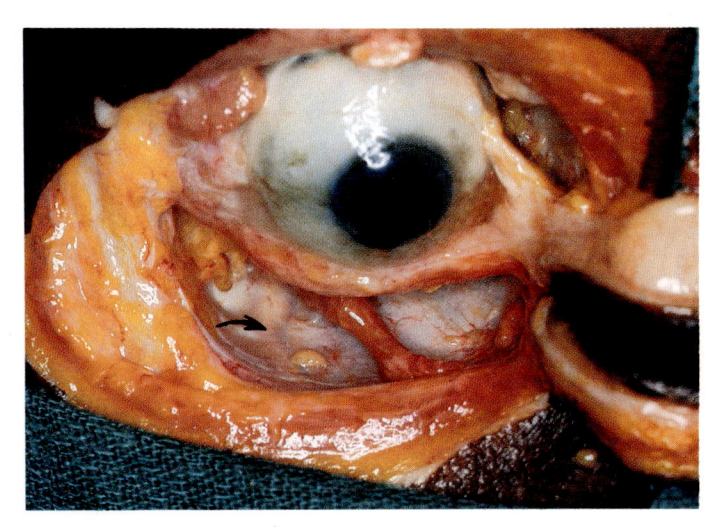

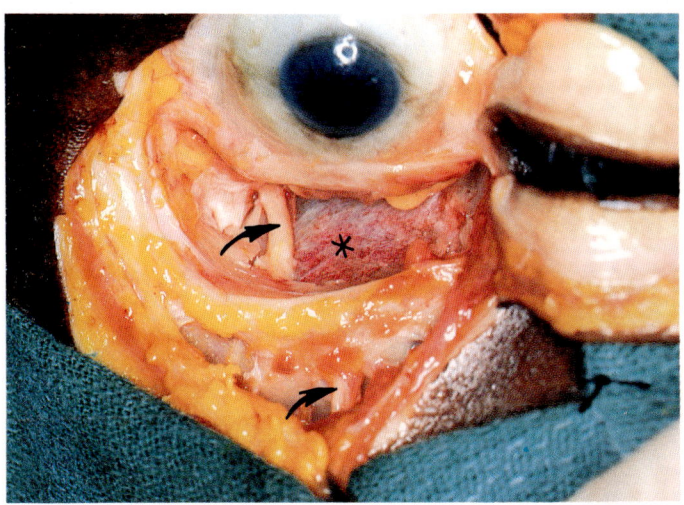

FIG. 3-19. Part of the bony floor of the orbit has been removed, exposing the maxillary sinus mucosa (*) and infraorbital nerve *(arrow)*. Note that the nerve courses from a lateral position to its more medially located infraorbital foramen on the anterior face of the maxilla.

FIG. 3-20. The infraorbital nerve is seen exiting from the infraorbital foramen. The foramen, approximately 4 mm in diameter, opens in an inferior or inferior and medial orientation. The foramen is approximately 7 to 10 mm below to the infraorbital margin. A needle directed to enter the foramen for a nerve block should be placed through the skin below the medial aspect of the nasolabial fold.

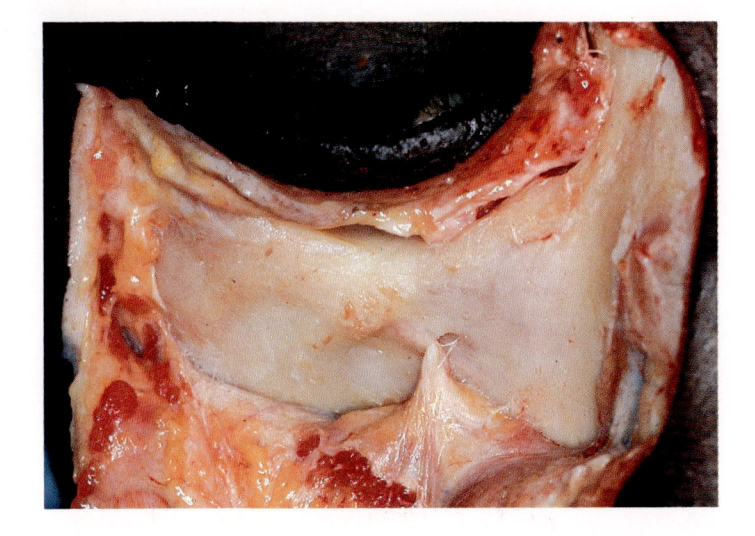

CHAPTER 3

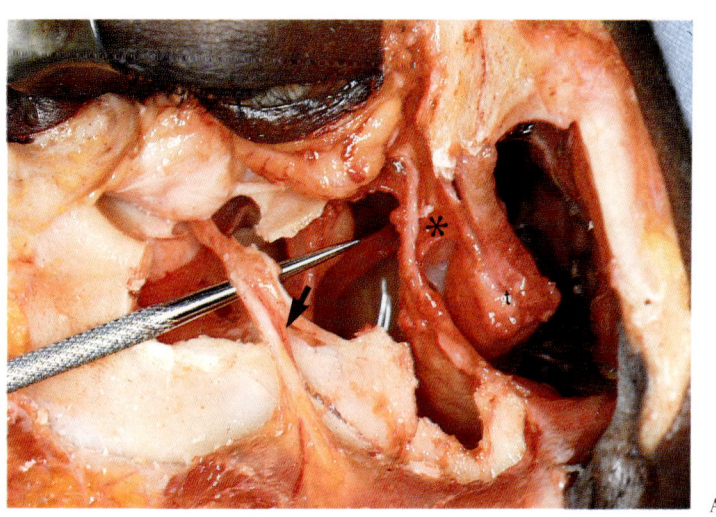

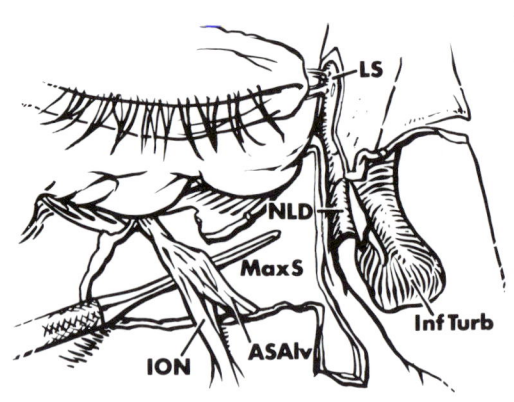

FIG. 3-21. A & B: A medial portion of anterior maxillary bone has been removed. The anterior superior alveolar nerve *(arrow)* branches from the infraorbital nerve 5 to 20 mm proximal to the foramen. It then travels along the inner surface of the maxilla or within a fine bony canal. This branch supplies sensation to the incisors and cuspid as well as the gingiva of the anterior alveolus. Note the nasolacrimal duct (*) and inferior turbinate (t). The duct empties into the inferior meatus approximately 4 cm from the alar base and 1.5 cm from the floor.

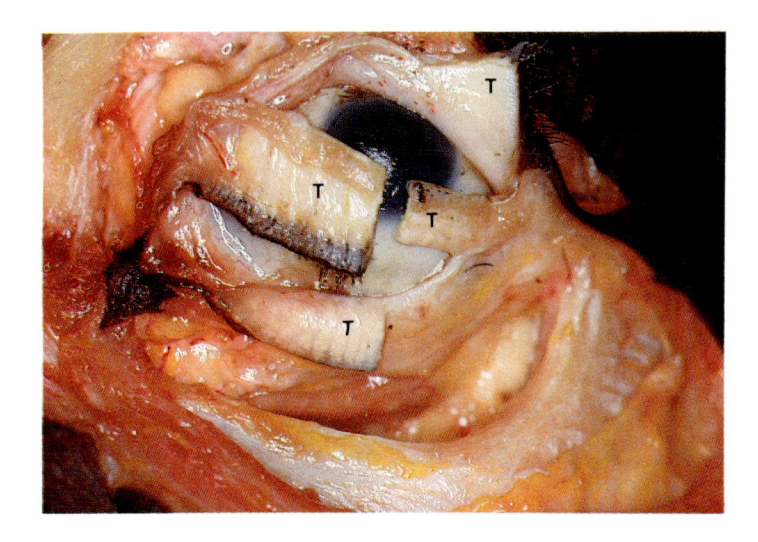

FIG. 3-22. In this dissection, the vertical height of the upper and lower lid tarsi (T) are compared. The tarsal plates provide skeletal support for the eyelids and consist of dense fibroelastic tissue and oil-secreting Meibomian glands. The glands can be seen running vertically within the tarsal plates. The height of the tarsal plate in the upper lid varies between 9 and 11 mm, whereas the lower lid tarsal plate measures between 3.8 and 4.5 mm in height.

4

Lacrimal Apparatus

The lacrimal apparatus consists of those structures involved with the production, distribution, and drainage of tears. Proper tear film maintenance protects the eyes and provides a refractive optimal surface.

CHAPTER 4

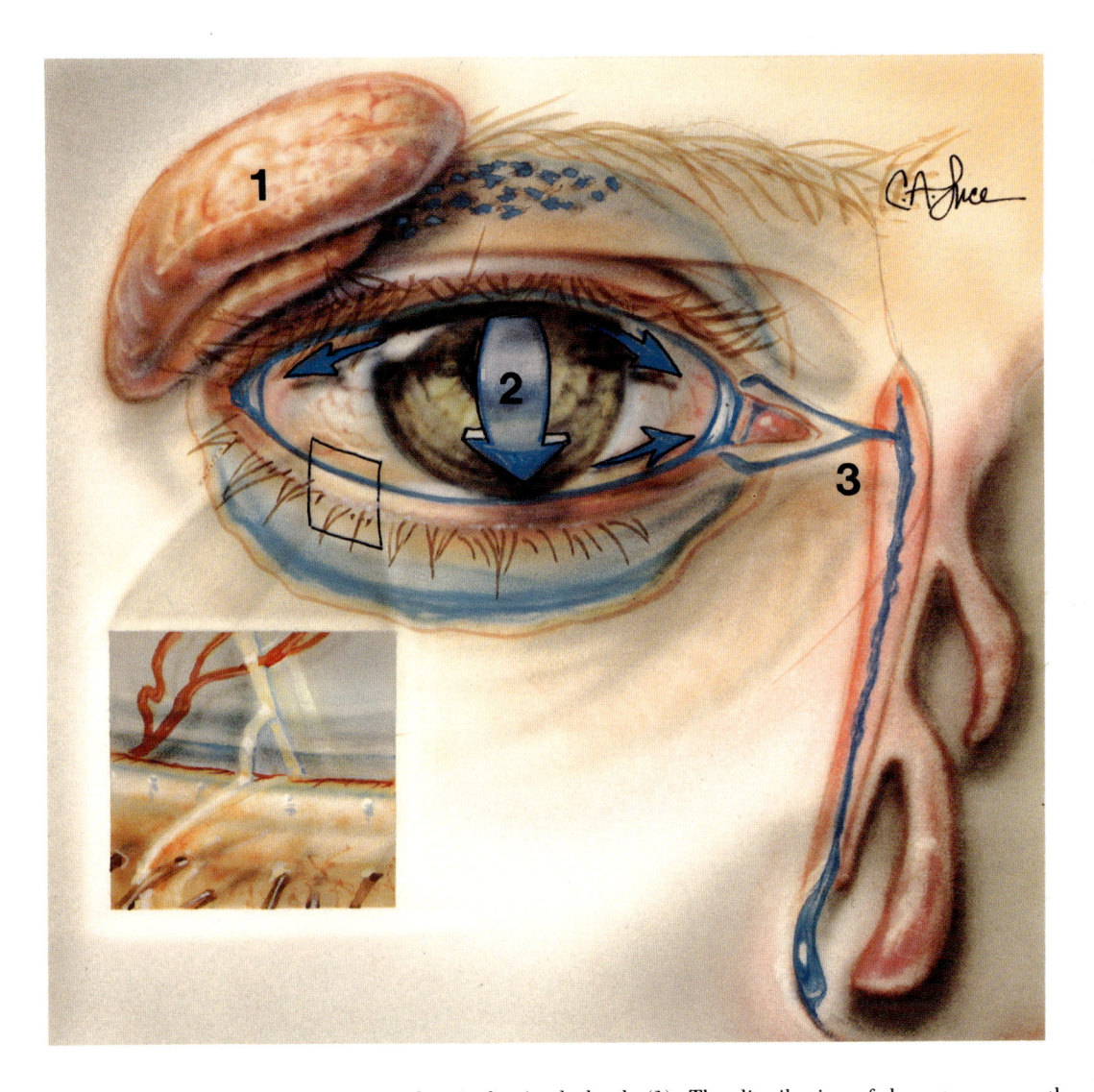

FIG. 4-1. Tears are produced by accessory and main lacrimal glands (1). The distribution of these tears over the surface of the eye is achieved by movements of the eyelids (2) performing a squeegee action of the marginal tear bead *(inset)* shown here in optical cross-section by a slit lamp beam. The passage of tears into the nose occurs via the lacrimal drainage system (3).

LACRIMAL APPARATUS

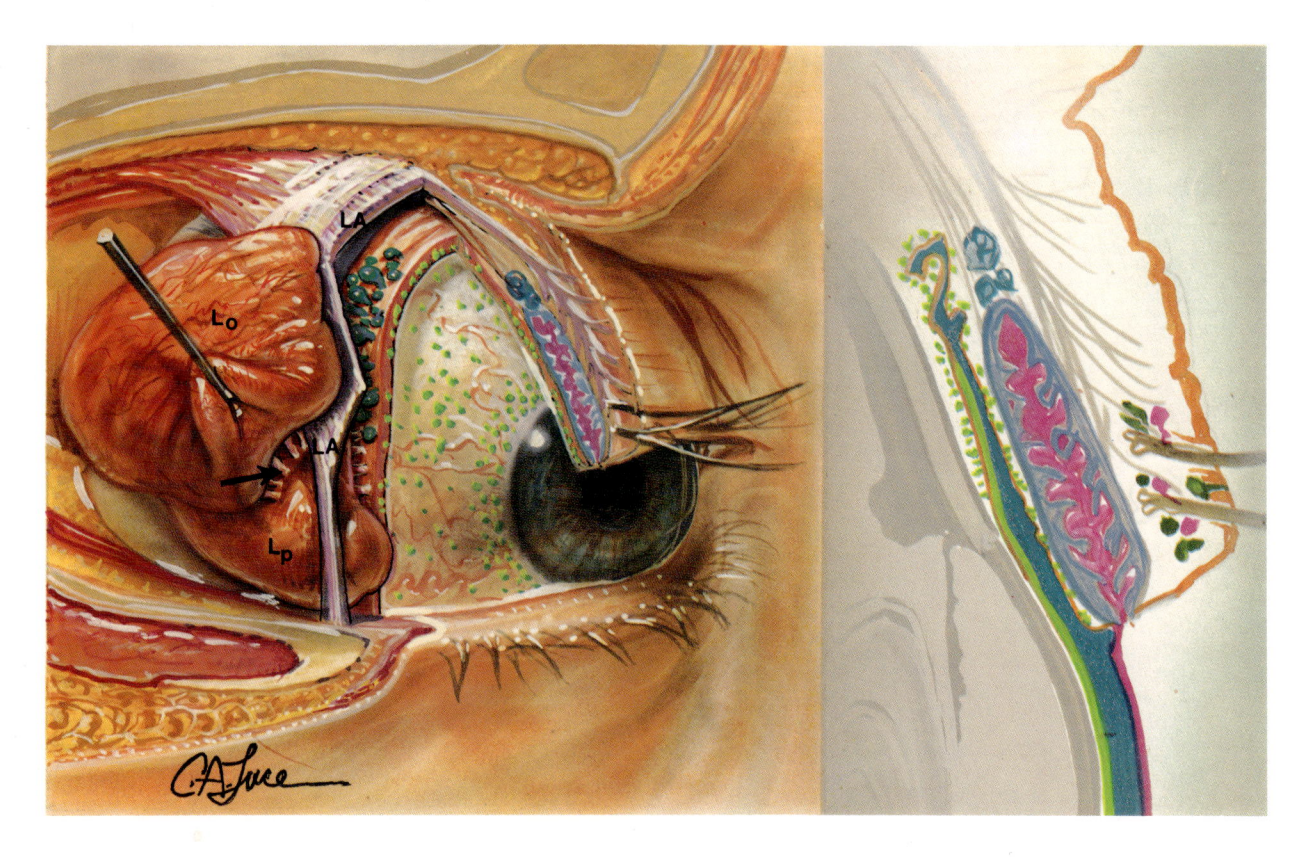

FIG. 4-2. The lacrimal secretory system controls the amount of tears and is divided into basic and reflex secretors. The basic secretors are composed of three sets of glands. The first set of basic secretors consists of the conjunctival, tarsal, and limbal mucin-secreting goblet cells, which produce a mucoprotein layer covering the epithelial surface of the cornea *(green)*. This is the inner layer of the precorneal tear film. The overlying aqueous layer is able to spread more uniformly because of this inner layer.

The second group of basic secretors is composed primarily of the accessory lacrimal exocrine glands of Krause and Wolfring, present in the subconjunctival tissues *(blue)*. These glands produce the intermediate aqueous layer of the precorneal tear film. The volume and thickness of this aqueous layer may be further augmented by tear output from the reflexly stimulated main lacrimal gland.

The third group of basic tear secretors consists of the oil-producing Meibomian glands (approximately 20 in each lid) and the palpebral glands of Zeis and Moll *(pink)*. These glands produce the outermost layer of the precorneal tear film. This superficial lipid layer helps stabilize the tear film and retards evaporation of the underlying aqueous layer. This three-layer film is distributed across the globe by normal apposition of lids to globe upon closure.

The reflexly-stimulated lacrimal gland is divided into two portions by the lateral horn of the levator palpebrae superioris (LA). The orbital lobe of the lacrimal gland (Lo) is considerably larger than the palpebral portion (Lp). The superior surface of the gland is convex and is connected to the frontal bone by weak trabeculae.

The smaller palpebral portion of the gland lies in the lateral part of the upper eyelid adjacent to the conjunctiva. The palpebral portion is approximately one-third the size of the orbital portion and can occasionally be seen in the superior lateral conjunctival fornix when the lid is everted. It may prolapse and be visible without lid eversion also.

The tear ducts *(arrow)* from the orbital portion traverse the palpebral portion. The palpebral gland empties its contents via 6 to 12 tear ductules into the superior lateral conjunctival fornix. Therefore, removal of the palpebral portion of the gland essentially blocks orbital lobe secretion to the conjunctival fornix.

Chapter 4

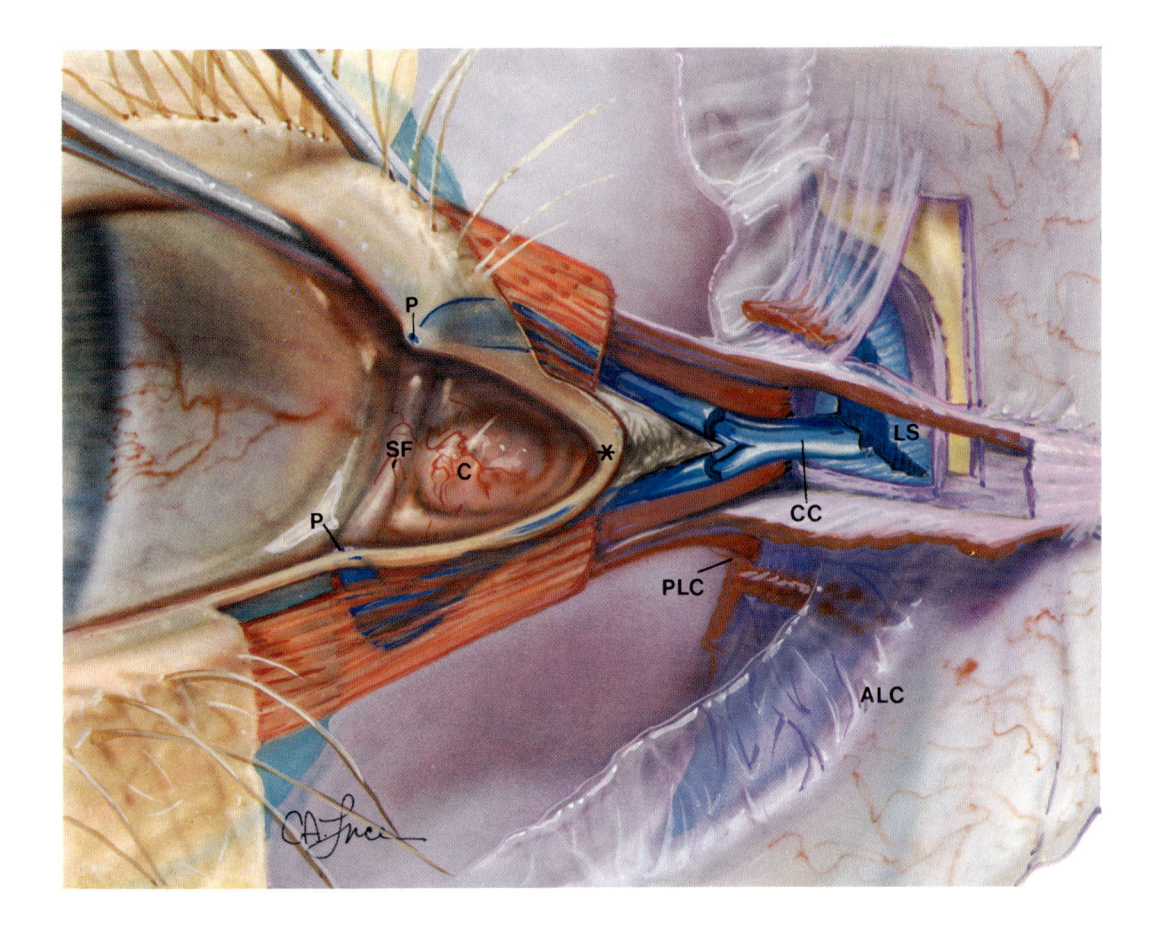

Fig. 4-3. The lacrimal drainage system. The caruncle (c) found medial to the semilunar fold (SF) consists of modified skin within which may be found sweat glands, goblet cells, and fine hair follicles. The upper and lower puncta (p) open 5 to 7 mm lateral to the canthal angle (*). The lower lid punctum is usually 1 to 2 mm more lateral than the upper. Each punctum opens at the apex of a whitish mound of tissue called the papilla.

The vertical portion of each canaliculus, the ampulla, measures approximately 2 mm. The ampulla of the canaliculus is a dilatation that occurs just prior to the transition to a horizontal direction. The punctal os is approximately 0.3 mm in diameter; however, the canaliculus may be 1 to 2 mm in diameter. The horizontal components measure approximately 8 mm and usually converge to form the common canaliculus (cc). However, these canaliculi may enter the lacrimal sac (LS) separately, approximately 3 to 5 mm from the apex, slightly behind the midlateral surface of the sac. The canaliculi are invested posteriorly by the deep heads of the pretarsal orbicularis oculi. Anteriorly the canaliculi are covered by fibers from the pretarsal orbicularis muscle and more medially by fibers of the medial canthal tendon.

The lacrimal sac (LS) is located within the lacrimal fossa in the medial orbital wall. It is ensheathed by an extension of periorbita and surrounding fascia. This so-called lacrimal fascia is especially thick and adherent superiorly. *En face*, the posterior lacrimal crest (PLC) is slightly (1–3 mm) more lateral than the anterior lacrimal crest (ALC).

LACRIMAL APPARATUS

FIG. 4-4. The movement of tears into the nose is thought to be assisted by an active lacrimal pump mechanism that is dependent on (a) the superficial and deep heads of the pretarsal orbicularis oculi muscles; (b) the deep heads of the preseptal orbicularis oculi muscle; and (c) the lacrimal diaphragm. With the eyelids open *(upper)*, the puncta lie in contact with the lacrimal lake, where the tears collect medially. The canaliculi remain patent as the lacrimal sac tends to collapse.

Upon eyelid closure *(middle)*, tears are milked lateral to medial. The deep heads of the pretarsal muscles contract, shortening the canaliculi and closing their ampullae. Simultaneously, the deep heads of the preseptal muscles, attached to the fascia of the sac (the lacrimal diaphragm), pull this fascia laterally creating a negative pressure within the sac.

As the lids reopen *(lower)*, the lacrimal diaphragm returns to its relaxed position, creating sufficient pressure to propel the tears into the nasolacrimal duct. The canaliculi reopen at this phase to allow collection of more tears. (See also Fig. 5-3.)

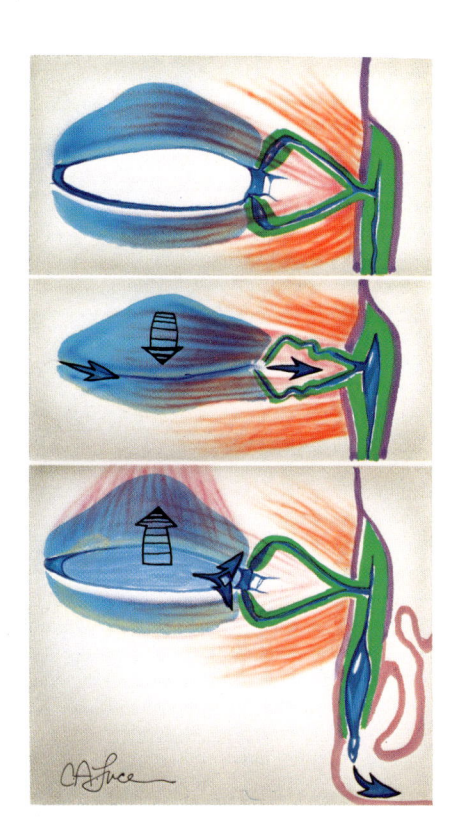

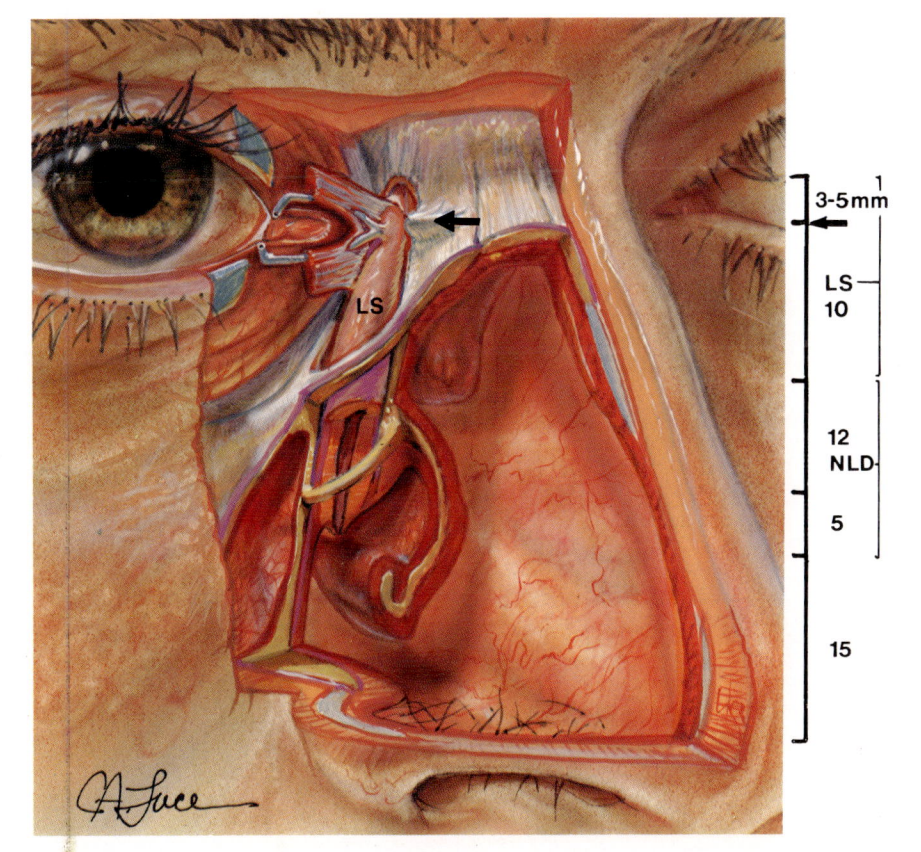

FIG. 4-5. The lacrimal sac is usually 15 mm in height, 3 to 5 mm of this extending superior to the medial canthal tendon *(arrow)*. The intraosseous portion of the nasolacrimal duct is much shorter than usually suspected; i.e., approximately 12 mm. The duct empties into the inferior meatus approximately 15 mm from the floor of the nose.

CHAPTER 4

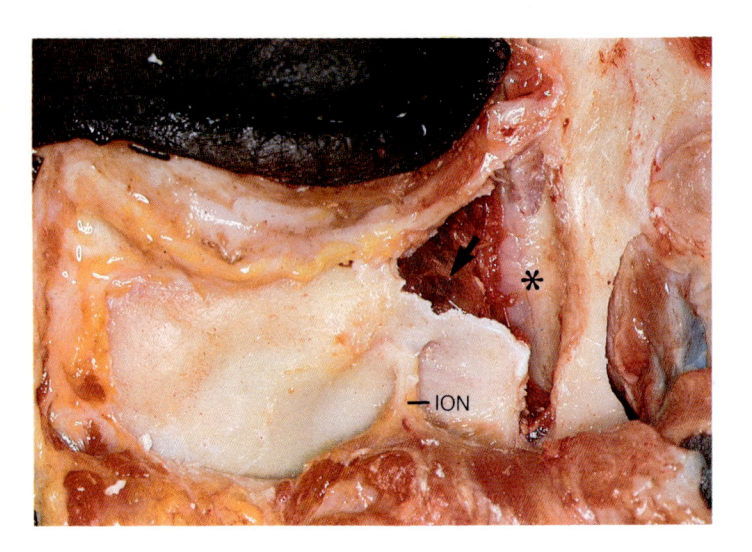

FIG. 4-6. The anterior maxilla has been cleared of muscle to expose the infraorbital nerve (ION). Maxillary bone removal medial and superior to the nerve exposes the underlying maxillary sinus *(arrow)* and the intraosseous portion of the nasolacrimal duct (*).

FIG. 4-7. The inferior turbinate is incised anteriorly *(blue arrow)* and reflected upward. The probe exits the slit valve (of Hasner) as noted, approximately 40 mm from the opening of the nose.

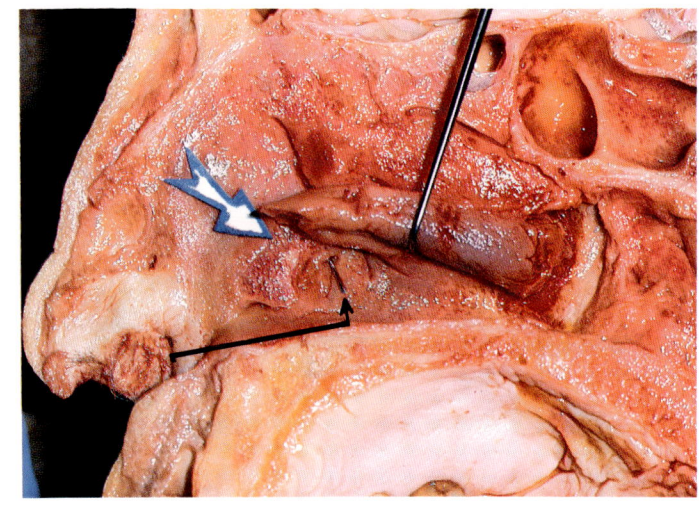

38

LACRIMAL APPARATUS

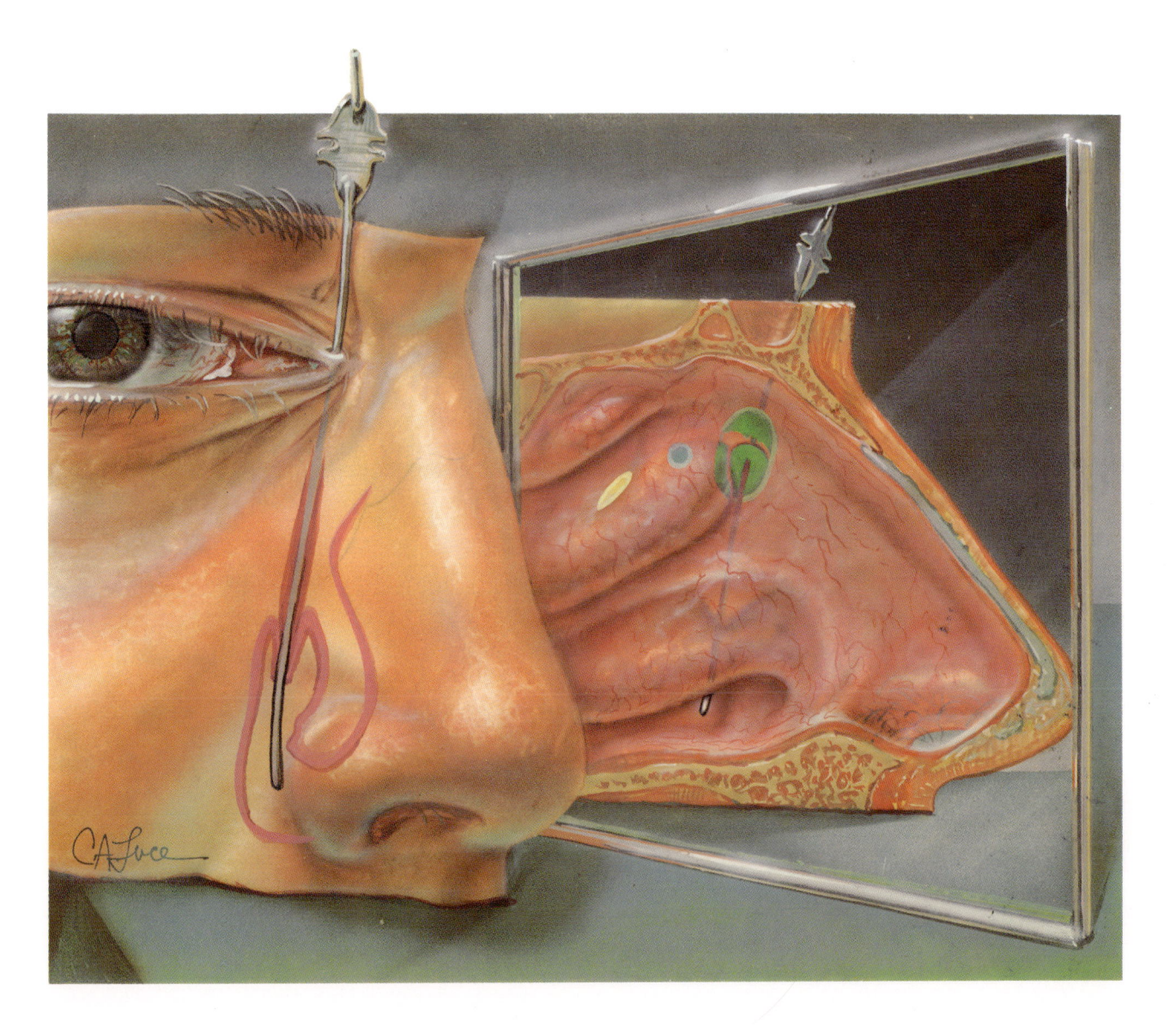

FIG. 4-8. The anterior tip of the middle turbinate corresponds well to the location of the lacrimal fossa *(green)*. The opening of the nasofrontal duct in the middle meatus *(blue)* and the ethmoidal ostium *(yellow)* are shown.

5
Medial Canthus

An understanding of the structures at the medial canthus allows the surgeon to reconstruct properly disinsertions of the medial canthal tendon with consideration toward the anterior, posterior, and superior components of its attachment.

Chapter 5

Fig. 5-1. The skin of the medial upper and lower lids and superior lateral nose is removed. Note the thinness of the orbicularis oculi fibers through which the underlying orbital septum and fat can be seen. A vertical orientation of some of the medial orbicularis fibers *(arrow)* is noted. This part of the muscle has been termed the depressor supercilii; i.e., that which pulls down the medial eyebrow. Imbedded in the muscle approximately 1 cm from the canthus (*) are the angular vessels (V), which continue superiorly to the midforehead region. The palpebral portion of the orbicularis oculi muscle diverges laterally from its origins at the medial canthal tendon and neighboring bone.

Fig. 5-2. The muscle fibers of the upper and lower superficial palpebral portions of the orbicularis oculi are reflected to expose the tendon (*). Note the angular veins *(arrow)* and the anastomotic connections. The anterior lacrimal crest lies under the vein. Although in this specimen the tendon does not seem to extend far into the frontal process of the maxillary bone, the full insertion is covered by soft tissue.

Fig. 5-3. The nose has been cut away to show the origins of the orbicularis oculi fibers and their relation to the lacrimal sac *(green)*. The anterior component of the medial canthal tendon *(arrow)* extends forward anterior to the sac. The palpebral portion of the orbicularis oculi muscle can be separated into pretarsal *(orange)* and preseptal *(red)* components. Furthermore, these components possess deep and superficial heads as they pass medially. The deeper fibers pass posteriorly to the lacrimal sac and its fascia and to the posterior lacrimal crest and are vital to proper lacrimal pump function. The deeper pretarsal fibers have been termed *Horner's muscle*, the *pars lacrimalis*, or *tensor tarsi*. Note that the medial canthal tendon extends beyond the anterior lacrimal crest (ALC) to the frontal process of the maxilla. The orbital portion of the orbicularis oculi fibers *(magenta)* arises from the medial orbital margin.

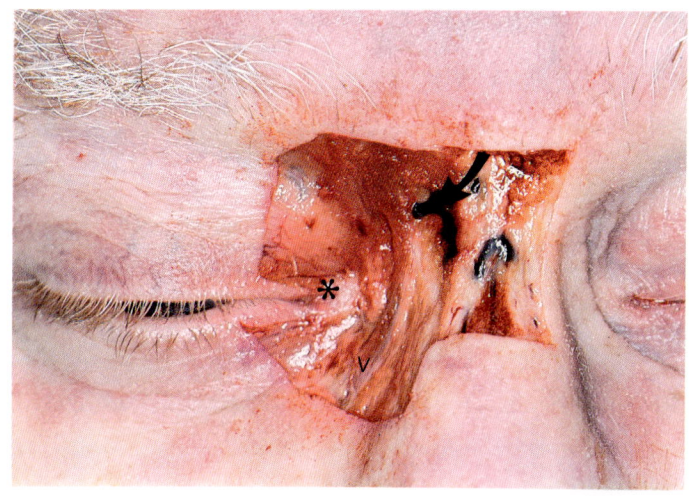

Fig. 5-1.

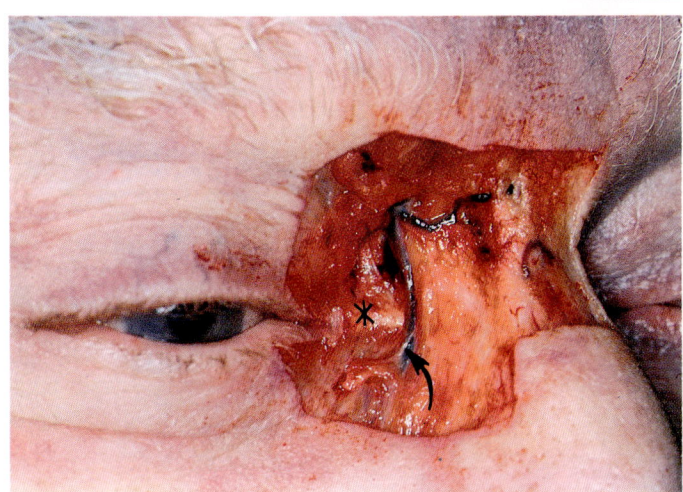

Fig. 5-2.

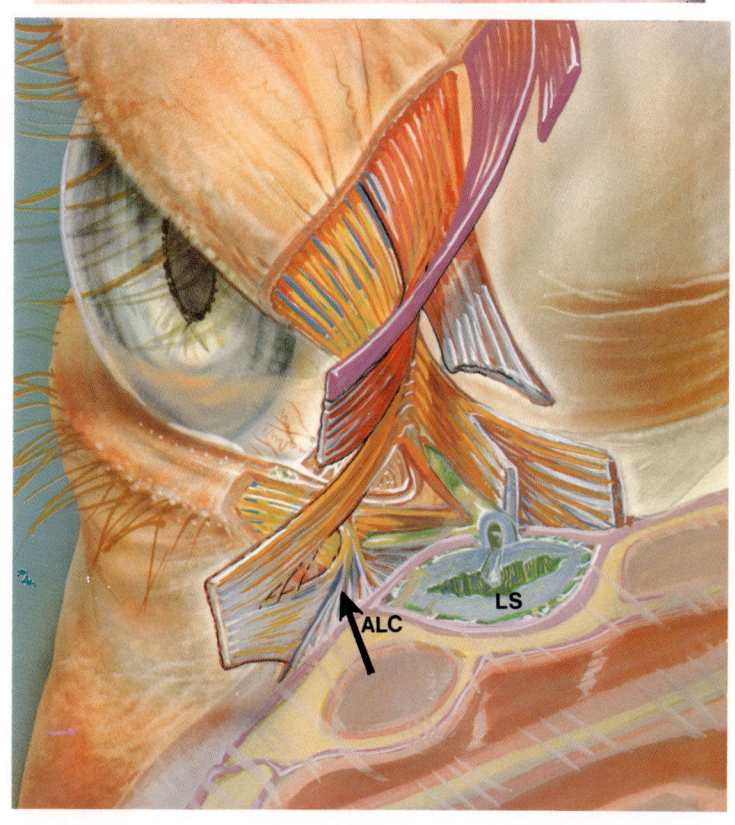

Fig. 5-3.

CHAPTER 5

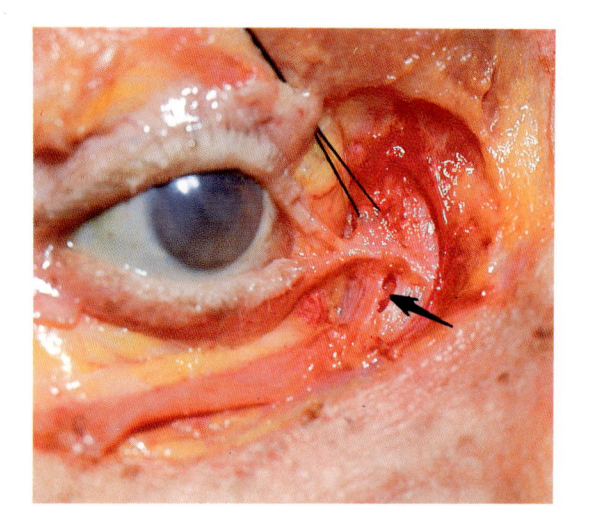

FIG. 5-4. The orbicularis oculi muscles have been dissected from the medial canthal tendon and surrounding bone. A small rent below the tendon exposes the inside of the inferior portion of the lacrimal sac *(arrow)*. Above the horizontal portion of the tendon, the fascia thickens over the upper lacrimal sac. A silk suture has been placed around this fascia, the so-called vertical component of the medial canthal complex.

FIG. 5-5. A closeup depicts the vertical fascial expansion *(black arrow)* of the medial canthal complex. The *red arrow* points to the edge of the uncovered lacrimal sac within the lacrimal fossa.

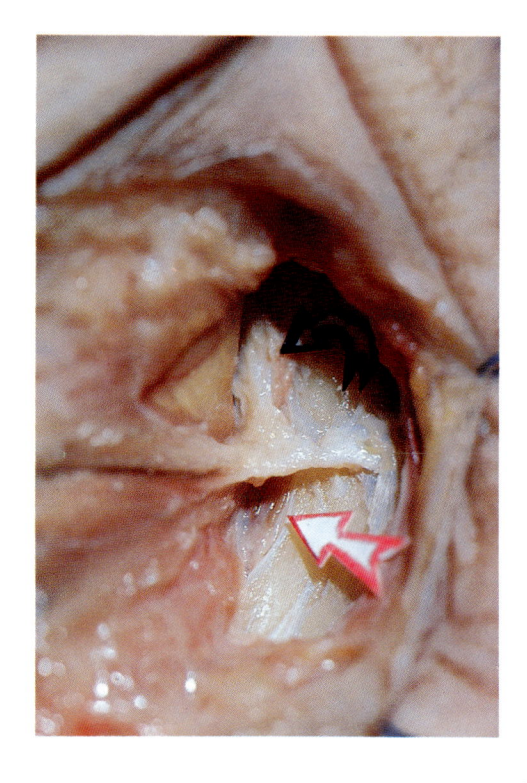

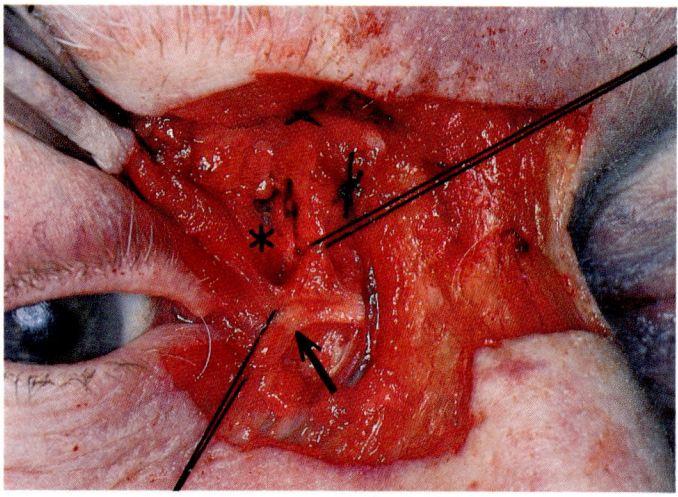

FIG. 5-6. A: A suture is placed at the canthus around the anterior component *(arrow)*. The superior suture surrounds the vertical fascial support. Note the deep head of the preseptal orbicularis passing toward the posterior lacrimal crest (*).

44

FIG. 5-6. B: The anterior component has been transected at the anterior lacrimal crest. Traction inferolaterally with the suture leads to minimal displacement of the tendon *(arrows)* from the bone. This is due to the residual support from the posterior and superior components.

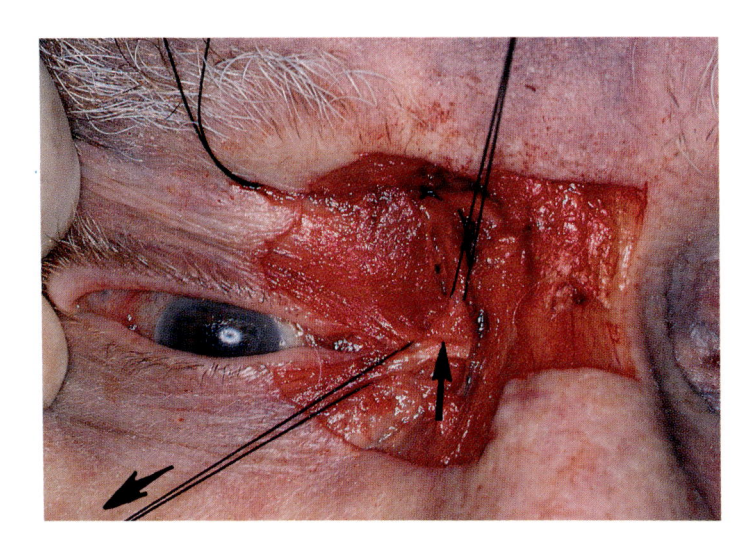

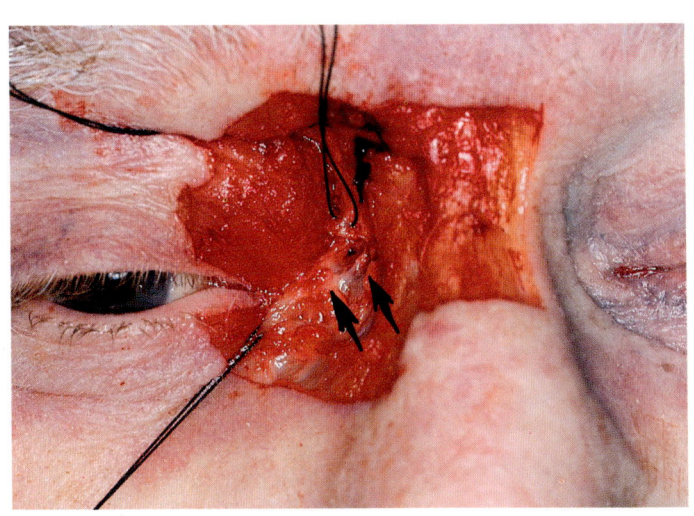

FIG. 5-6. C: The superior component has now been transected in addition. Distraction of the tendon end increases *(arrow)*. The telecanthus becomes more obvious.

FIG. 5-6. D: If all components of the medial canthal mechanism are released, the dystopia and telecanthus are increased. In this specimen, even the posterior components, i.e., deep heads, have been removed from the bone.

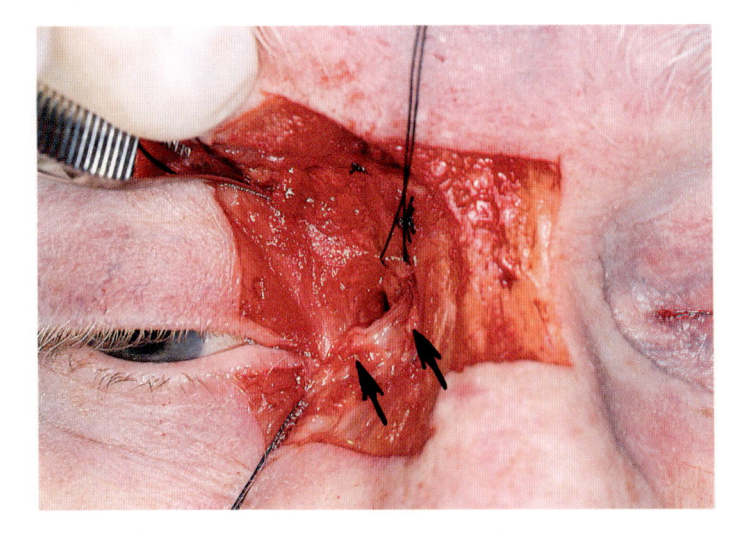

CHAPTER 5

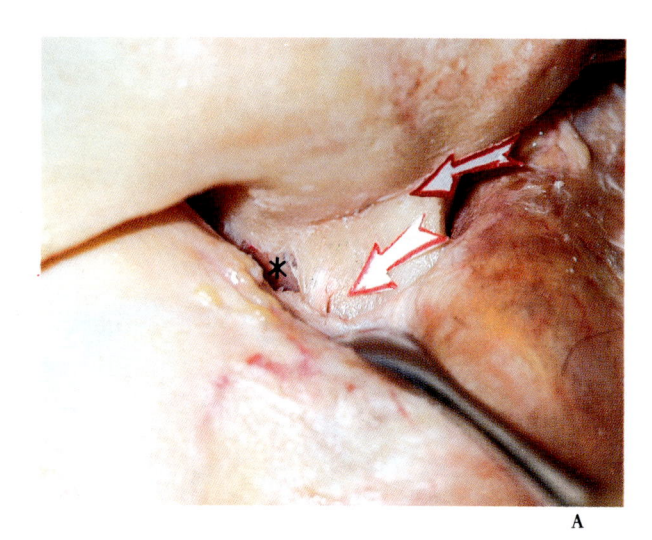

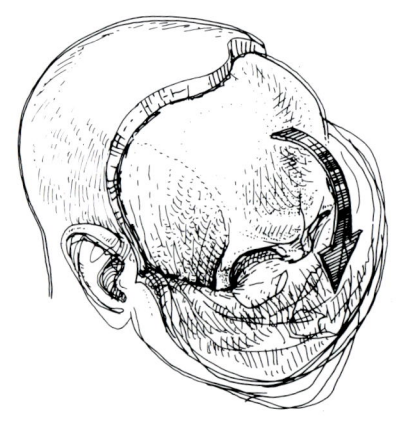

A

B

FIG. 5-7. A & B: Subperiosteal dissection via a bicoronal incision (scalp flap) provides access to the medial canthal region. The *upper arrow* depicts the nasofrontal suture, which may vary in position. The *lower arrow tip* rests 2 mm anterior to the vertical fascial component of the medial canthal complex. The lamina papyracea has been broken to expose the ethmoid labyrinth (*).

6

Lateral Retinaculum

Familiarity with the structure and function of the components of the lateral retinaculum is essential for a lateral surgical approach to the orbit.

CHAPTER 6

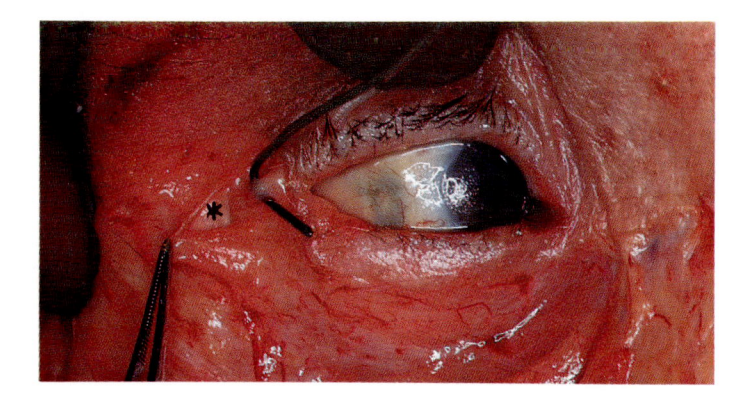

FIG. 6-1. The orbicularis oculi muscle has been cut transversely to expose the periosteum over the lateral orbital rim (*) as well as the lateral canthal tendon. A probe may be noted below the lateral canthal tendon, which measured 2 to 2.5 mm wide and 6 to 7 mm long. It is not a very dense structure. The tendon actually splits. One leaf continues anteriorly in close association with the periosteum over the lateral orbital rim. The posterior element inserts on the lateral orbital tubercle (of Whitnall) approximately 5 mm behind the rim.

FIG. 6-2. The lateral canthal tendon is further exposed. Debate exists regarding whether or not the orbital septum passes in front of or behind this structure. Controversy continues also as to whether this tendon arises from the orbicularis oculi muscle, submuscular fascia, tarsal plates, or some combination of these elements.

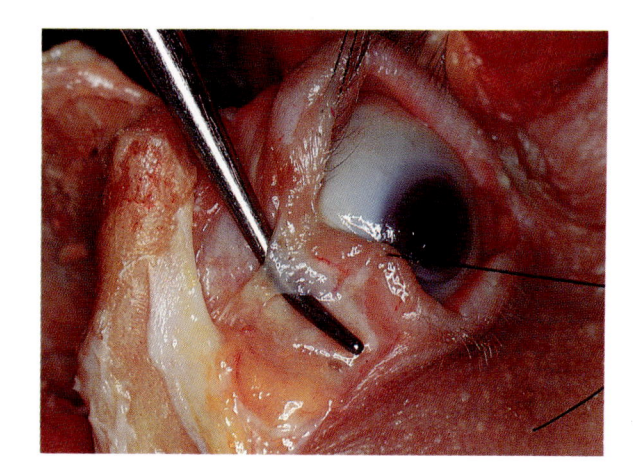

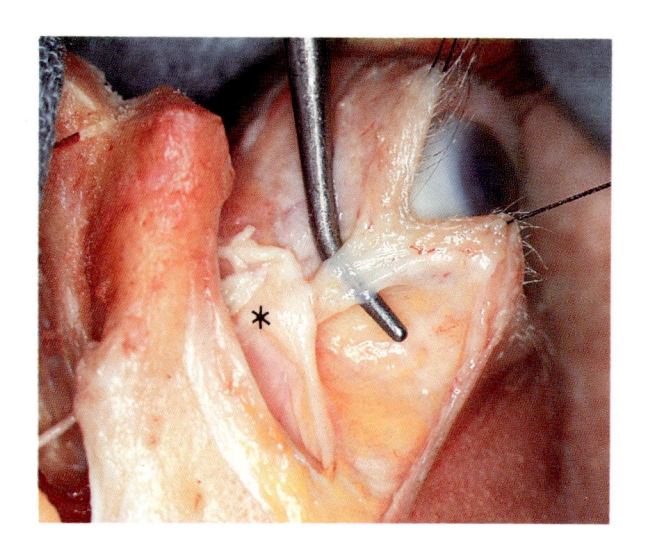

FIG. 6-3. The periosteum has been elevated from the lateral orbital rim and from the area of the lateral orbital tubercle. A definite thickening of the periorbita is noted in this area (*).

48

LATERAL RETINACULUM

FIG. 6-4. The bony lateral orbital rim has been excised to expose the thickened periorbita (×) at the region of the lateral retinacular complex. The forceps support the lateral canthal tendon, the most anterior component of the lateral retinaculum. This specimen exhibits a rather thick tendon.

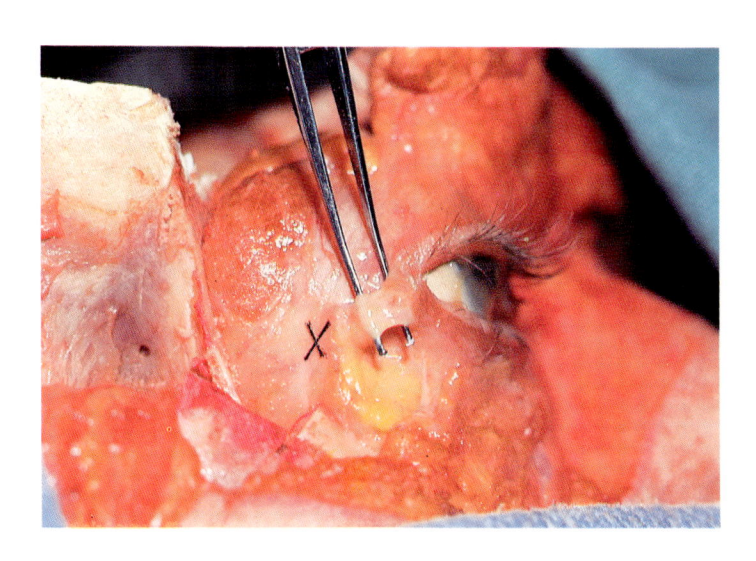

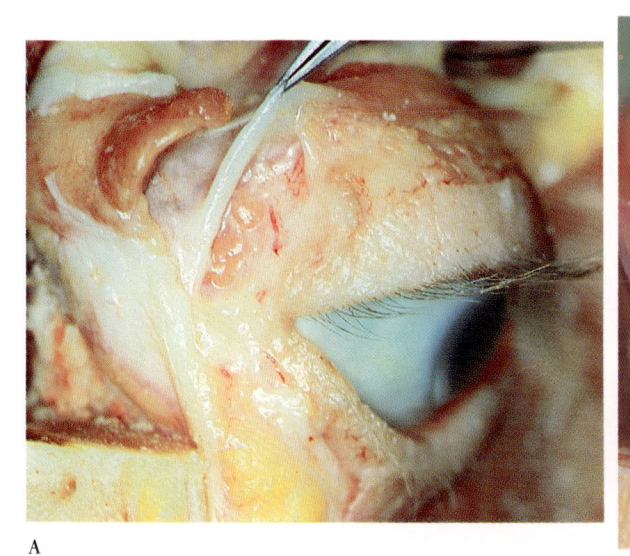

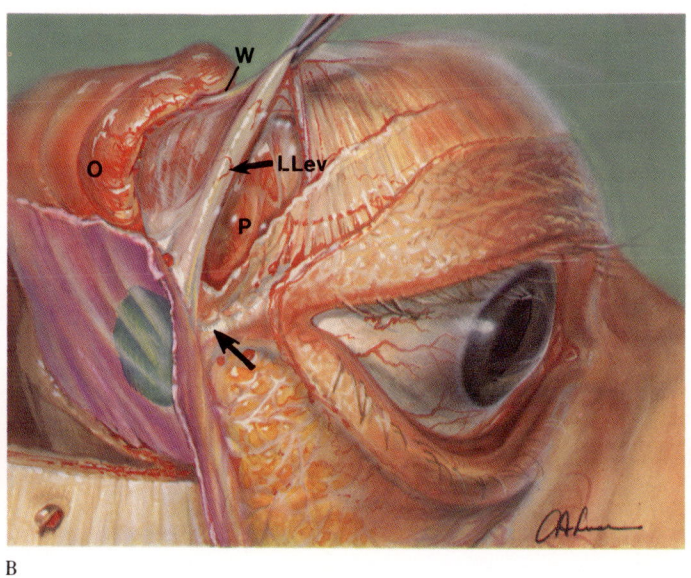

A

B

FIG. 6-5. A & B: The lateral horn of the levator aponeurosis *(arrow)* splits the lacrimal gland into its orbital (O) and palpebral (P) lobes. The lateral portion of Whitnall's ligament (W) inserts into the orbital lobe of the gland by way of the interglandular fascial septi. The inferolateral pole of the lacrimal gland usually rests at the level of the insertion of the lateral retinaculum *(green)*. The lateral retinacular structures which insert into the green shaded area are 1) the lateral horn of levator aponeurosis (LLev); 2) the lateral canthal tendon *(arrow)*; 3) the inferior suspensory ligament (Lockwood); and (4) the check ligament of lateral rectus muscle. (See Figs. 8-7 and 8-8.)

Chapter 6

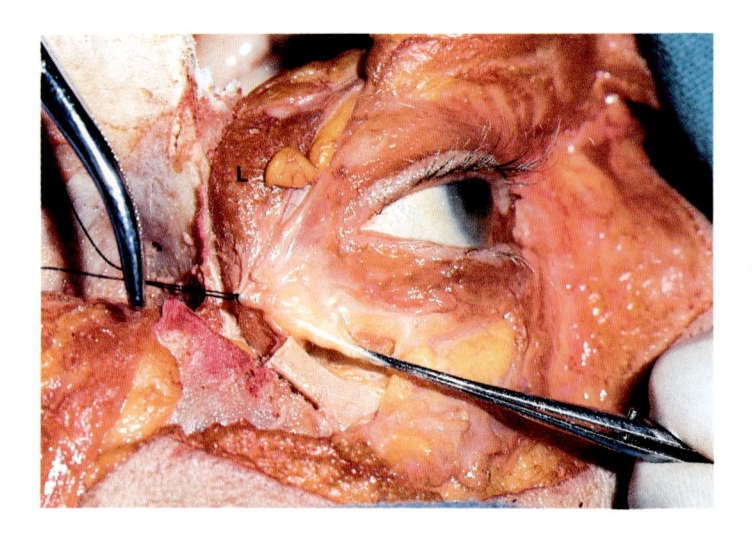

Fig. 6-6. A suture is placed at the area of insertion of the lateral retinaculum. The forceps demonstrate the lateral anterior portion of the inferior suspensory ligament of Lockwood, which thus forms part of the lateral retinaculum. Note the extent of the lacrimal gland (L). The entire ligament of Lockwood may be perceived better by reviewing Figs. 3-16 and 8-8.

Fig. 6-7. The bone of the lateral orbital rim has been removed as in a lateral orbitotomy. An incision made in the periorbita exposes the lacrimal gland (L) with its lacrimal artery. The lacrimal gland is lifted to expose the underlying lateral rectus muscle (LR). At the anterior portion of the lateral rectus muscle, the check ligament *(arrow)* may be seen coursing toward the lateral retinaculum. This is better seen in Fig. 8-7.

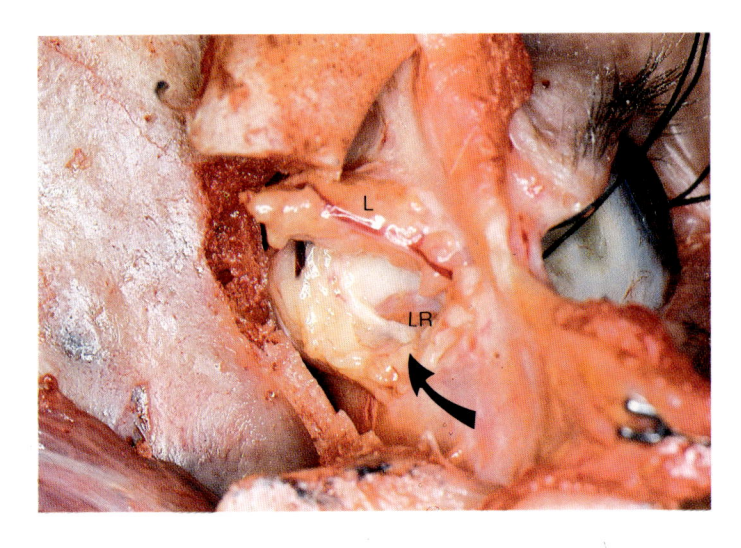

7

Orbital Dissection

Chapter 7

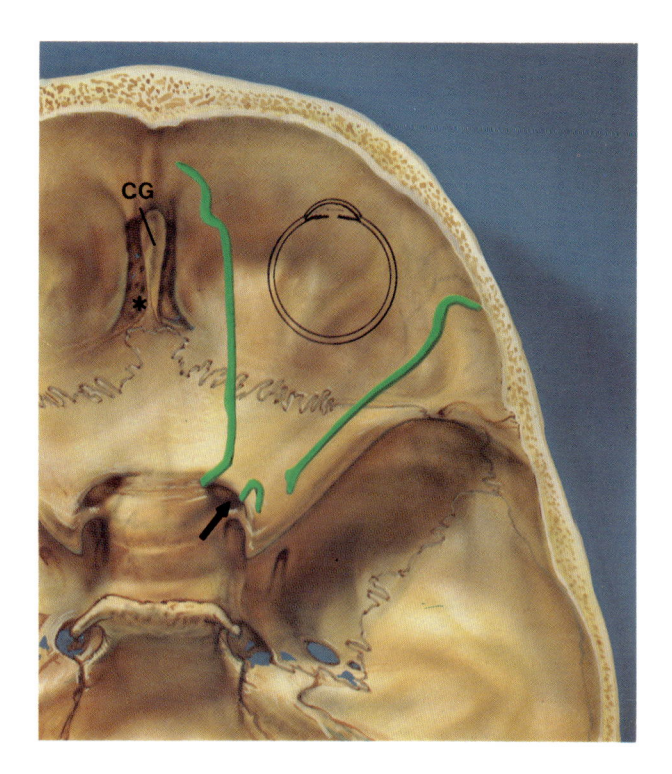

Fig. 7-1. The calvaria has been removed. The dura mater, which lines the anterior cranial fossa, has been removed. Note the cribriform plate (*) and the midline crista galli (CG). The roof of the orbit is formed primarily by the orbital plate of the frontal bone, which may be divided by the frontal sinus. The limits of the medial and lateral orbital walls are outlined in *green*. The optic nerve enters the orbit via the optic canal *(arrow)* within the lesser wing of the sphenoid bone. The relative position of the globe is shown.

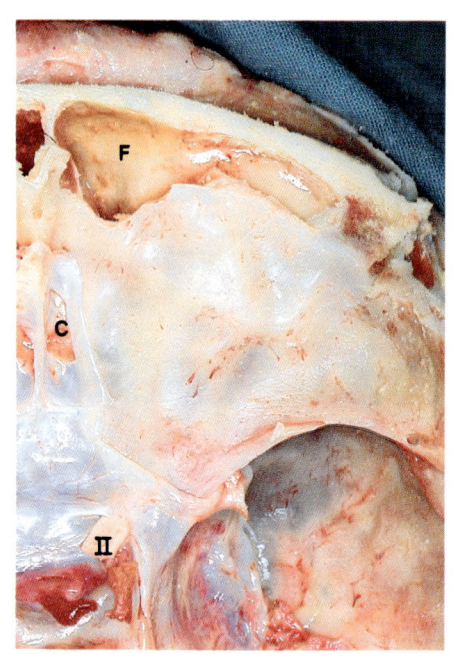

Fig. 7-2. The extent of the frontal sinus (F) varies from person to person. The cribriform plate (C) and optic nerve (II) are noted. The roof of the orbit, thin in spots, is intact.

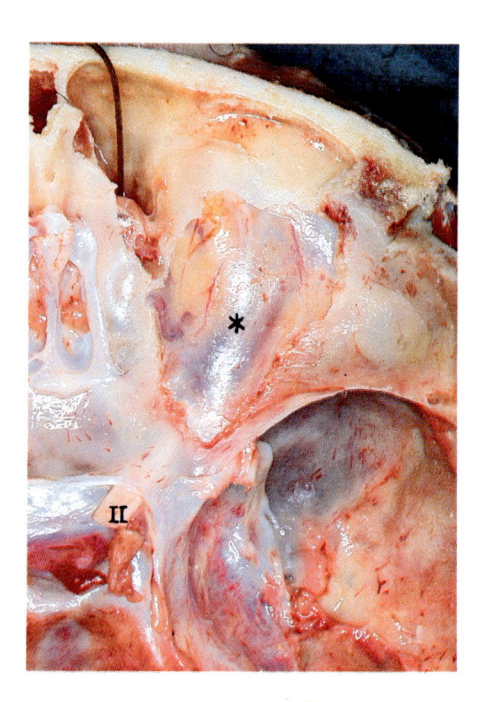

Fig. 7-3. The bony orbital roof has been removed to expose the underlying periorbita (*). Note the optic nerve (II) entering the apex of the orbit through the optic canal. A probe enters the nasofrontal duct.

52

ORBITAL DISSECTION

FIG. 7-4. Within the cranial cavity, the optic nerve is surrounded only by the pia mater (p) and measures approximately 10 mm. At the entrance to the optic canal, the arachnoid and dura are added to the coverings of the optic nerve. The intracanal portion of the nerve is 9 to 10 mm. At the exit of the optic canal, the dura splits into two layers: the outer layer continuous with the periorbita and the inner layer forming the dural covering of the optic nerve. Thus, within the orbit and canal, the nerve is surrounded by dura, arachnoid, and pia. The orbital portion of the optic nerves is approximately 30 mm before entering the sclera (1 mm). The ophthalmic artery (OA) originates from the internal carotid artery (ICA) to travel with the optic nerve in its sheath to exit the dura at the anterior end of the canal. Most often, the ophthalmic artery courses laterally.

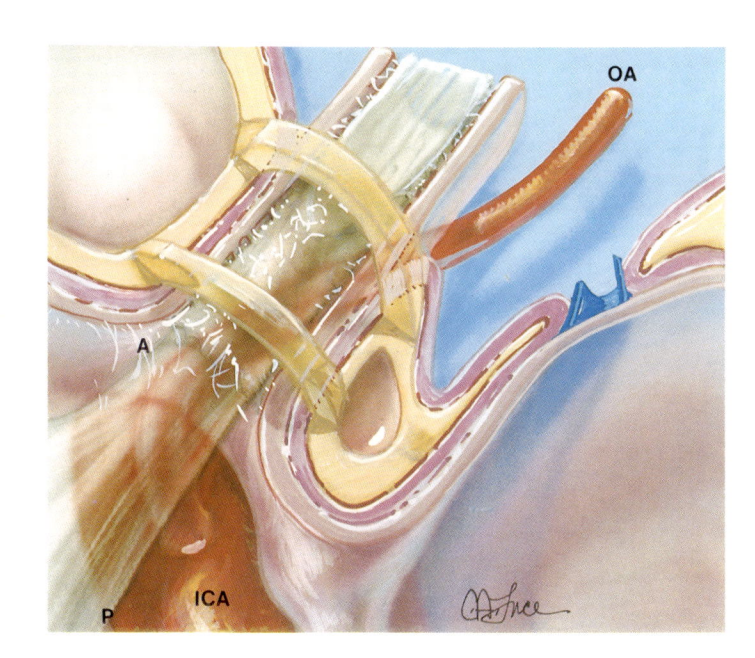

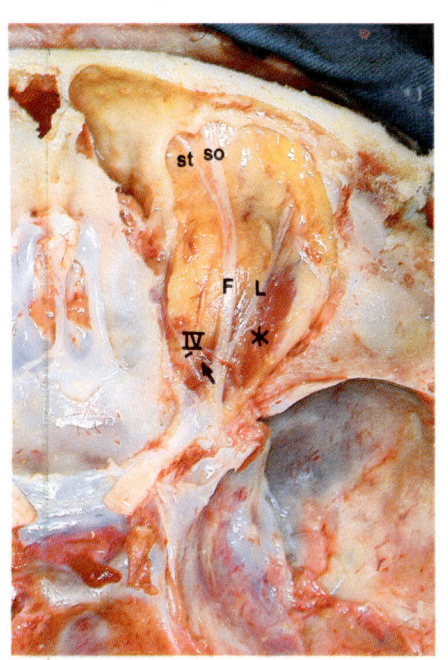

FIG. 7-5. The periorbita has been removed to reveal the most superior structures of the orbit, which are the nerves. The ophthalmic division of the trigeminal nerve enters the orbit via the superior orbital fissure. This nerve divides into three sensory branches: lacrimal (L), frontal (F), and nasociliary (not shown). The frontal nerve, which is the largest of these branches, enters above the annulus between the lacrimal (L) and the trochlear (IV) nerves. The lacrimal nerve, the smallest branch, is noted coursing temporally but medial and parallel to the lateral rectus muscle (*). The frontal nerve lies on the levator palpebrae muscle *(arrow)* and then divides anteriorly into supraorbital (so) and supratrochlear (st) branches. The deeper nasociliary branch is not seen at this level.

FIG. 7-6. At the apex of the orbit, the trochlear nerve (IV) enters the proximal third of the superior oblique muscle (SOb). The trochlear nerve enters the orbit via the superior orbital fissure above the annulus with the frontal nerve (F). The trochlear nerve divides into three or four branches that supply the superior oblique muscle. The levator palpebrae muscle (Lev) is again noted below the frontal nerve.

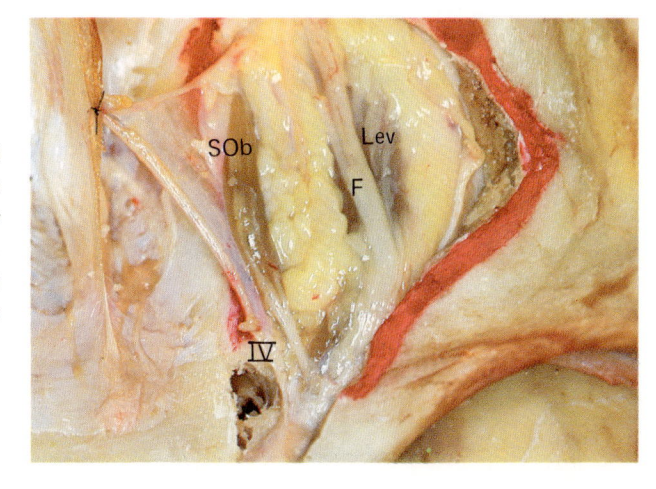

Chapter 7

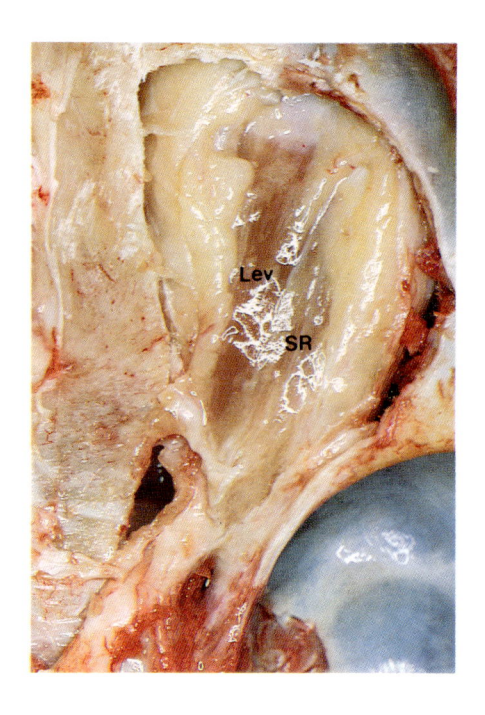

Fig. 7-7. The frontal and lacrimal nerves, as well as some orbital fat, have been removed. The levator palpebrae muscle (Lev) arises from the periorbita of the lesser wing of the sphenoid superior to the annulus and progresses forward. The edge of the superior rectus muscle (SR) is noted as it courses forward to insert onto the globe.

Fig. 7-8. The superior oblique muscle *(clamped)* is reflected medially, exposing the nasociliary nerve (N). This nerve passes through the superior orbital fissure within the annulus. It courses medially above the optic nerve and below the superior rectus muscle. The first division of the nasociliary nerve is the posterior ethmoidal nerve (of Luschka), which passes through the posterior ethmoidal foramen to provide sensation to the posterior ethmoidal sphenoid sinuses. It is often absent, as in this dissection. The nasociliary nerve usually divides at the region of the anterior ethmoidal foramen into its terminal branches: the anterior ethmoidal nerve (*) and the infratrochlear nerve (IT). The anterior ethmoidal nerve passes between the superior oblique muscle (SOb) and the medial rectus muscles, leaving the orbit via its foramen. This nerve supplies the anterior and middle ethmoidal sinuses and a portion of the frontal sinus. The nerve enters the anterior cranial fossa at the level of the cribriform plate where it occupies an intracranial but extradural course. It then passes forward to exit the "nasal slit" in the cribriform plate. The nerve reaches the roof of the nose, providing sensation to the septum and lateral nasal wall. Its terminal branch, the dorsal nasal nerve, exits from the edge of the nasal bone to supply sensation to the tip of the nose (see Fig. 1-16A).

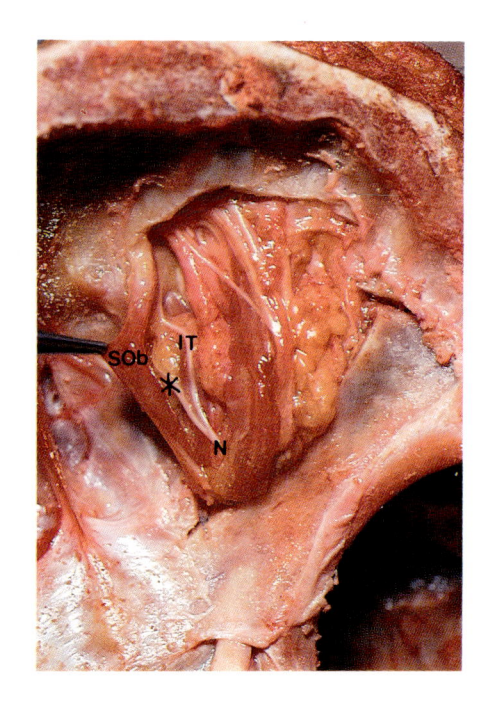

54

ORBITAL DISSECTION

FIG. 7-9. The periorbita (P) is fixed medially. A suture retracts the levator palpebrae muscle (Lev) laterally. Note the branches of the superior division of the oculomotor nerve *(arrow)* entering the levator muscle. The branches to the levator muscle either pierce the superior rectus muscle (*) or curl around its medial border, as demonstrated here. The superior oblique muscle (SOb) arises from the orbital apex at the junction of the medial wall and the roof of the orbit.

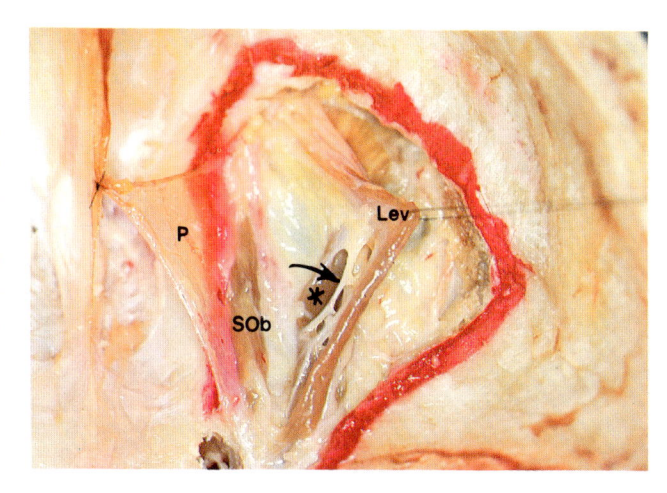

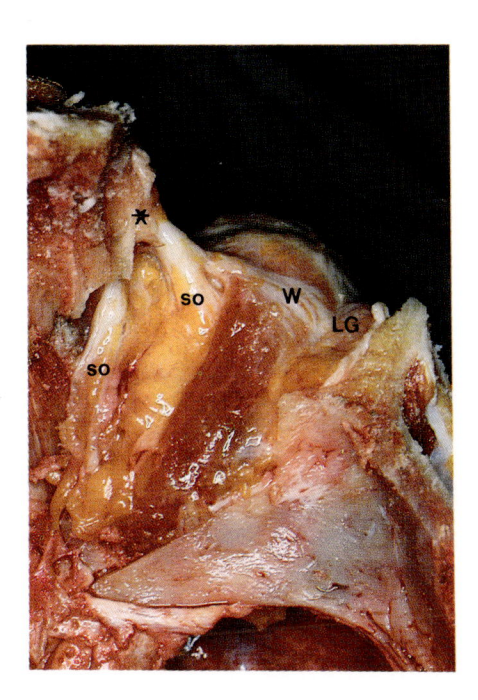

FIG. 7-10. The supraorbital bony bar has been removed from the lacrimal gland (LG) to the trochlea (*). The post-trochlear tendinous portion of the superior oblique muscle makes an angle of approximately 56° to the pretrochlear portion prior to insertion into the globe beneath the superior rectus muscle. Note the levator palpebrae muscle and the condensation of the fascia, Whitnall's ligament (W), coursing across the muscle.

FIG. 7-11. The levator palpebrae muscle (Lev) has been transected and flipped forward. A scalpel handle is noted in the upper conjunctival fornix (*). The superior rectus muscle *(small arrow)* overlaps the tendinous insertion of the superior oblique muscle (SOb). Some of the medial wall of the orbit has been removed to expose the anterior ethmoidal air cells (E). Note also the medial component of Whitnall's ligament (W) extending toward the trochlear apparatus.

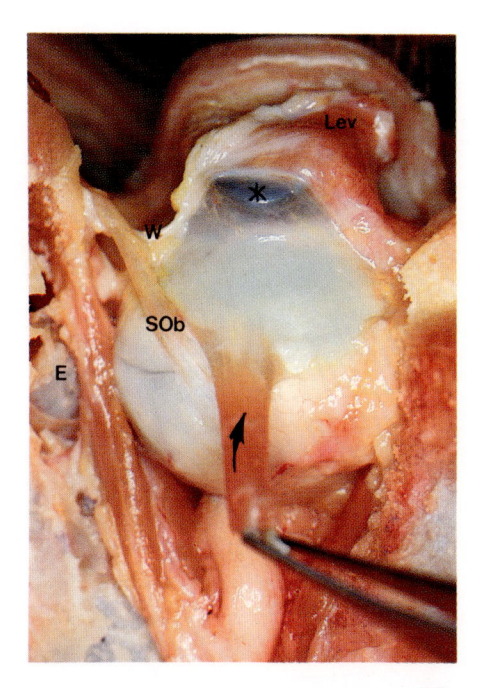

CHAPTER 7

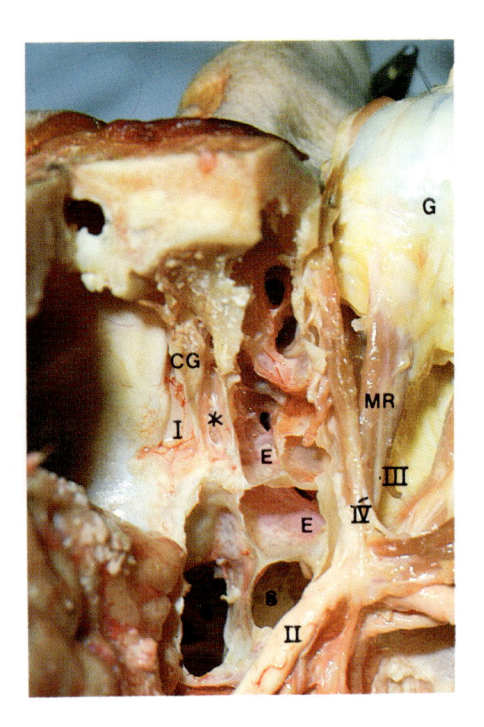

FIG. 7-12. The bony roof of the sphenoid sinus (S) and that of the ethmoid sinus (E) have been removed. Note the cribriform plate (*) and crista galli (CG). The distal portion of the olfactory bulb and nerve (I) is noted overlying the cribriform plate on the left side. The bony roof of the optic canal has been removed to demonstrate the course of the optic nerve (II). Note the trochlear nerve (IV) as it enters the posterior portion of the superior oblique muscle. The fat and vessels have been cleared to expose the medial rectus muscle (MR) subjacent to the superior oblique muscle. A branch of the inferior division of the oculomotor nerve (III) enters the medial rectus muscle at its posterior third. The globe (G) has been externally rotated to expose the medial rectus muscle more clearly.

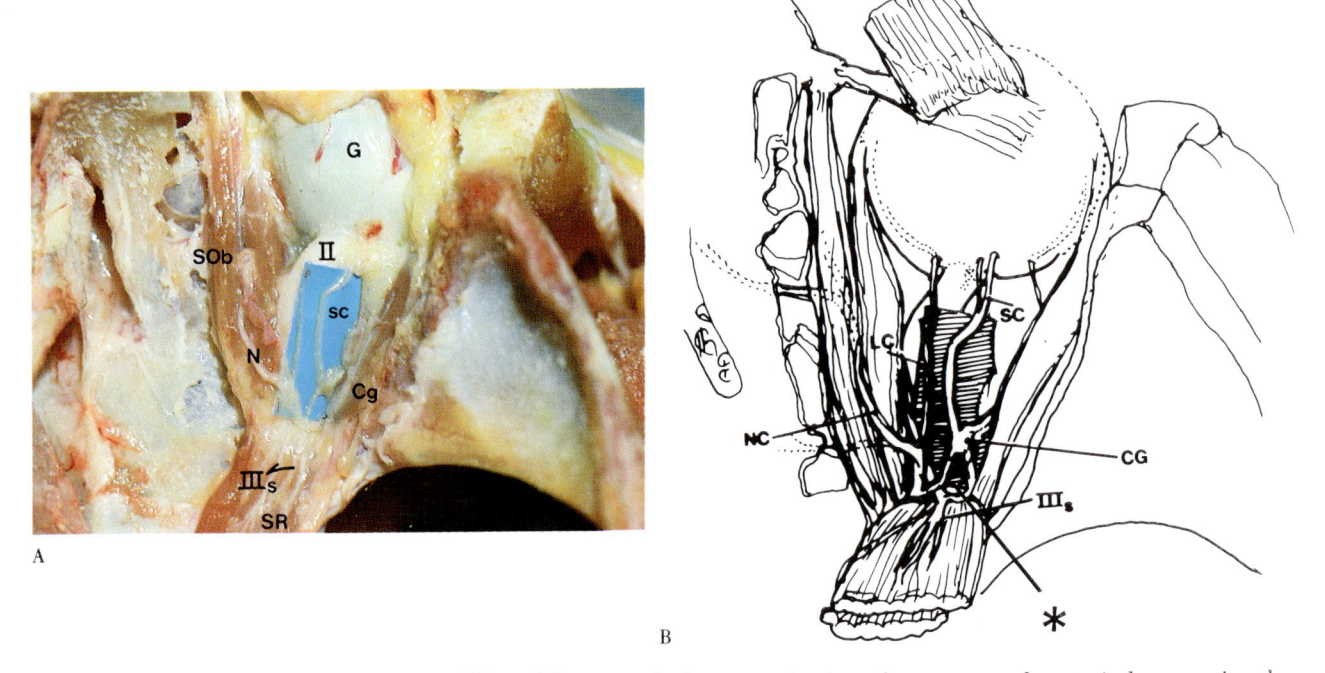

FIG. 7-13. A & B: The superior rectus (SR) and levator palpebrae muscles have been retracted posteriorly, exposing the superior division branches of the oculomotor nerve (IIIs) entering the muscles. The nasociliary nerve (N) inclines medially toward the superior oblique muscle (SOb). The optic nerve (II) is noted under the blue mat. A sensory ramus (*) leaves the nasociliary nerve to enter the ciliary ganglion (Cg). One (usually 2 or 3) of the long ciliary nerves (lc) is noted coursing forward to enter the globe (G), passing between the choroid and sclera. These nerves supply sensory fibers to the iris, cornea, and ciliary muscle and some sympathetic fibers to the dilator pupillae. One of the short ciliary nerves (sc), which may be 6 to 10 in number, passes forward from the ganglion to the sclera around the optic nerve.

ORBITAL DISSECTION

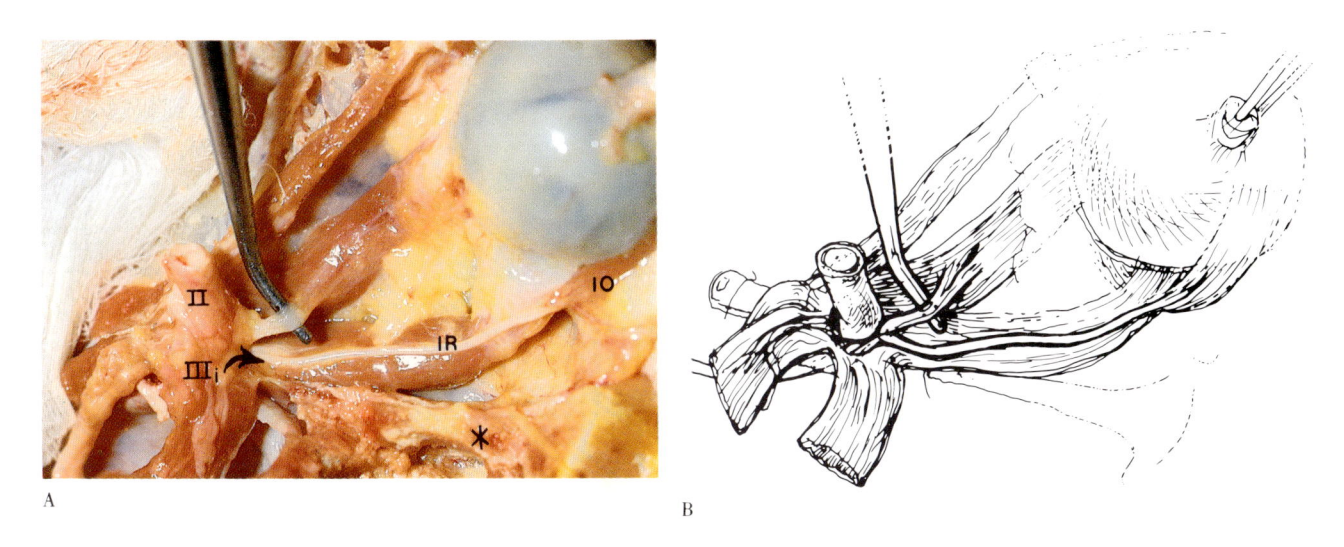

FIG. 7-14. A & B: Lateral view. The lateral orbital wall (*) has been removed. The superior rectus muscle, lateral rectus muscle, and optic nerve (II) have been transected and turned back. The inferior division of the oculomotor nerve (IIIi) immediately divides into three branches after passing through annular ring. The probe elevates the branch to the medial rectus muscle. The second branch *(arrow)* can be seen below this, piercing the junction of proximal and middle third of the inferior rectus muscle (IR). The nerve to the inferior oblique muscle (IO) continues along the orbital floor or alongside the inferior rectus muscle (IR) prior to piercing the inferior oblique muscle.

FIG. 7-15. The optic nerve (II) has been cut, and the globe (G) has been turned forward. Note the medial rectus muscle (MR) and nasociliary nerve (N) lying upon it. The inferior rectus muscle (IR) courses forward with the nerve to the inferior oblique (IO) lying on it. The lateral rectus muscle (LR) with its motor nerve (VI) is noted. The oculomotor nerve (III) travels in the lateral wall of the cavernous sinus, which has been unroofed. It then splits into its superior and inferior divisions just prior to entering the superior orbital fissure. The oculomotor nerve supplies all the extrinsic eye muscles except the lateral rectus and superior oblique muscles and also innervates the pupillary sphincter and the ciliary muscle. Note the trigeminal nerve (V) divisions. The abducens nerve (VI) is noted medial and inferior to the oculomotor.

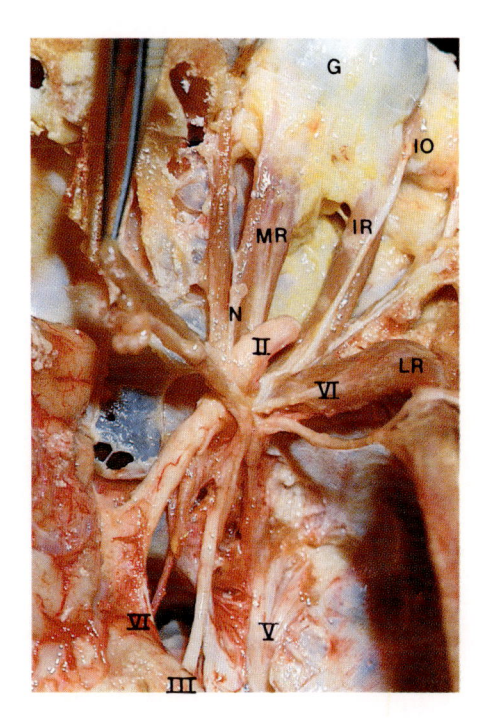

8

Extraocular Muscles and Associated Fascial Structures

The movement of the ocular globe is controlled by the extraocular muscles. A fascial system within the orbit supports the globe, limits ocular movements, and provides an interconnected scaffolding from one structure to another.

Chapter 8

Fig. 8-1. A fibrous thickening of the periosteum *(blue)* from which the recti muscles originate has been termed the annulus of Zinn, or common tendinous ring. The superior origin of the lateral rectus muscle (LR) separates the superior orbital fissure into two compartments. The portion of the orbital apex enclosed by the annulus is called the oculomotor foramen through which pass both divisions of the oculomotor nerve, the abducens nerve, and the nasociliary nerve. Those structures passing into the orbit laterally and outside the muscle cone or ring are the lacrimal, frontal, and trochlear nerves, ophthalmic vein, and a communicating branch off the middle meningeal artery. Note the optic nerve (II) as it passes through the lesser sphenoid wing lateral to the origin of the medial rectus muscle (MR). The inferior rectus muscle (IR) and superior rectus muscle (SR) origins complete the common tendinous ring. The superior oblique muscle *(arrow)* originates outside the annulus and superomedial to it. The levator muscle arises at the orbital apex superior to the superior rectus origin and thus outside the annulus. Because the superior and medial recti closely approximate the optic nerve, retrobulbar neuritis may be reflected in painful motility of these muscles.

Fig. 8-2. The course and relative positions of the extraocular muscles are shown from a superior orbital view. They are color coded according to their respective cranial nerve supply: (1) *(red)* oculomotor nerve (III), superior division: superior rectus muscle, levator muscle, and medial rectus muscle. (2) *(purple)* oculomotor nerve (III), inferior division: inferior rectus muscle and inferior oblique muscle. (3) *(green)* trochlear nerve (IV): superior oblique muscle. (4) *(blue)* abducens nerve (VI): lateral rectus muscle. Note that the inferior oblique muscle originates from the periosteum lateral to the nasolacrimal canal *(arrow)*.

The functions of the extraocular muscles are the following: Lateral rectus muscle: abduction. Medial rectus muscle: adduction. Inferior rectus muscle: primary, depression; secondary, adduction and extorsion (*extorsion* means that the superior pole of globe moves laterally); retraction of lower lid. Superior rectus muscle: primary, elevation; secondary: adduction and intorsion (*intorsion* means that the superior pole of globe moves medially). Superior oblique muscle: primary, depression; secondary, abduction and intorsion. Inferior oblique muscle primary: elevation; secondary, abduction and extorsion.

The vascular supply to the extraocular muscles occurs principally from the ophthalmic artery with some contribution from the lacrimal and infraorbital arteries. Each rectus muscle is supplied by two anterior ciliary arteries, except the lateral rectus, which has one. The anterior ciliary artery continues forward to penetrate the sclera at the muscle insertion, thus nourishing the anterior segment of the eye.

Extraocular Muscles

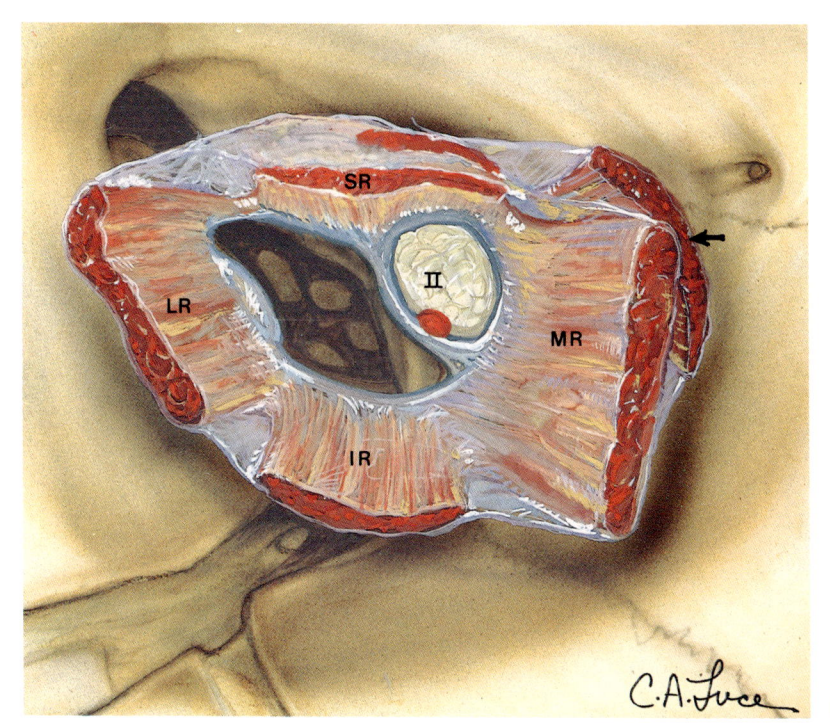

Fig. 8-1.

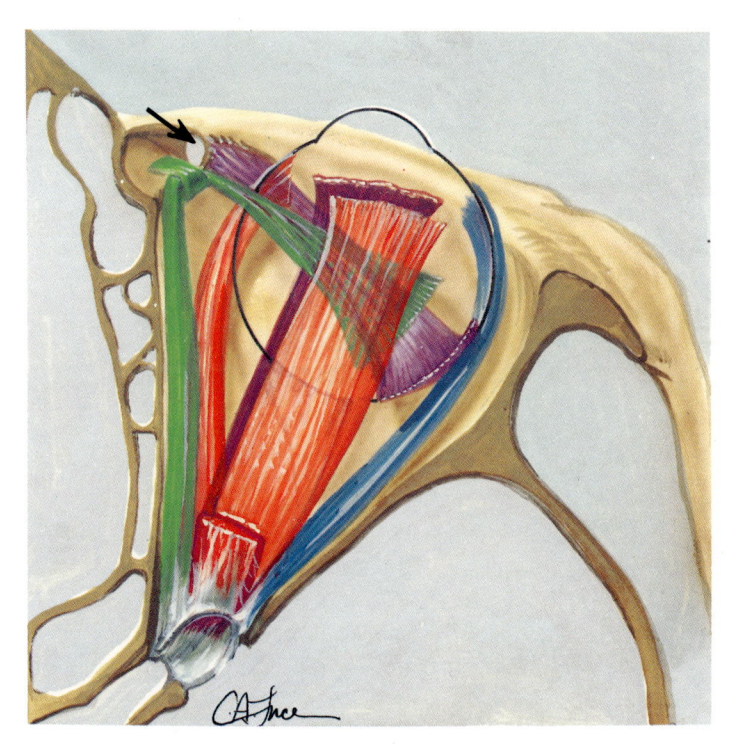

Fig. 8-2.

61

Chapter 8

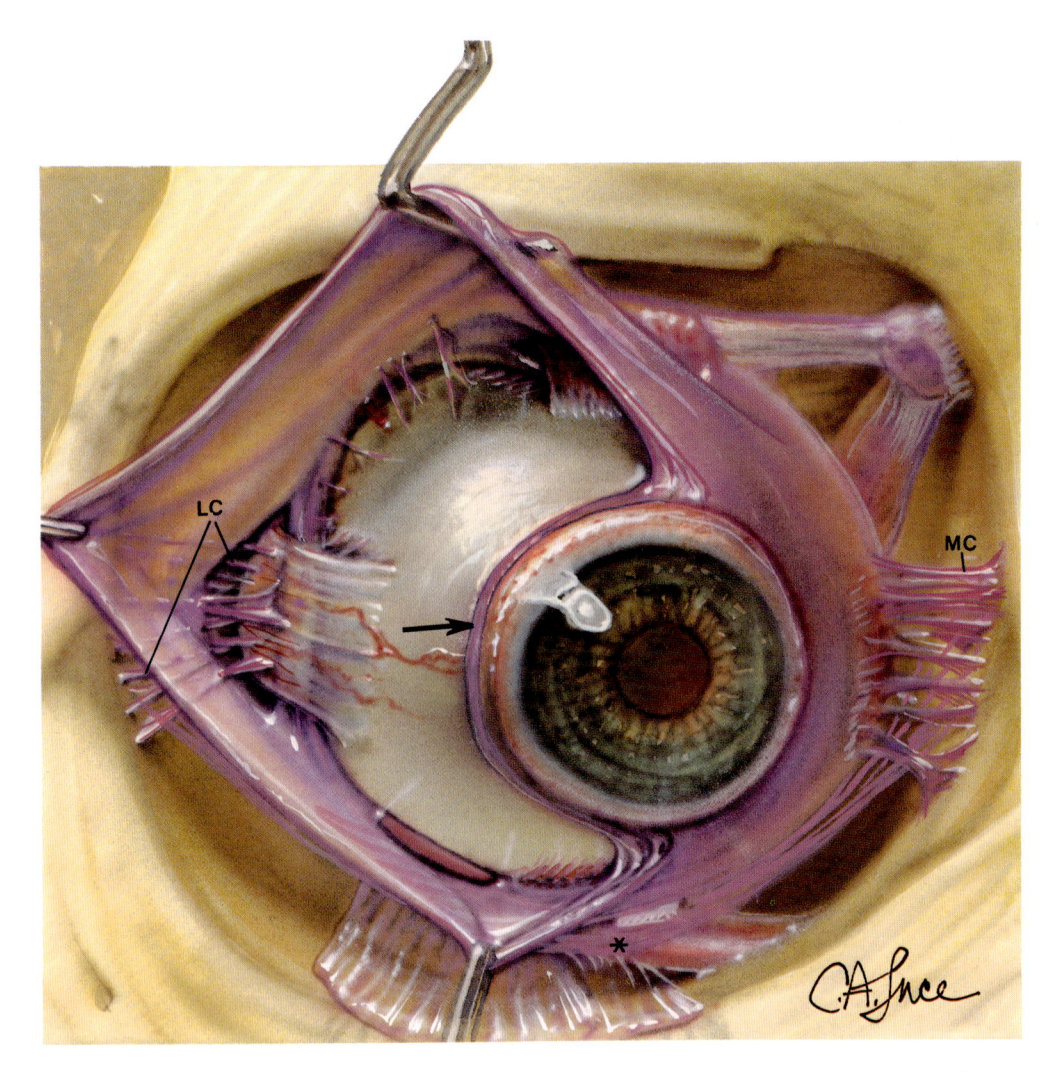

Fig. 8-3. The fascial framework of the orbit has classically been described as comprising (1) the bulbar fascia (Tenon's capsule); (2) fascial sheaths surrounding the extraocular muscles; (3) the intermuscular fascial septa; and (4) the medial and lateral check ligaments. More recently (Koornneef, 1977 a,b; 1979; 1982)[1], the fascial system has been described as tripartite: (1) Tenon's capsule and the fascia around the extraocular muscles; (2) connective tissue network connecting Tenon's capsule to the anterior periorbita; and (3) the diffuse fascial connections from the extraocular muscles to the posterior periorbita (unimportant). This recent classification may more easily explain the restrictive ocular phenomena that occur with orbital fractures.

Tenon's capsule, or the fascia bulbi, the dense fibroelastic layer that surrounds the globe, is elevated and retracted by hooks. The cut margin *(arrows)* is noted at the lateral limbus. The extraocular muscles must penetrate this fascia to insert on the globe. The intervening fascial network between the muscles (better seen in Fig. 8-4) is called the intermuscular septa. The anterior portion of the intermuscular septa is thick, providing an anatomic barrier in the front of the orbit. Of clinical importance for dissection: Tenon's capsule is tightly adherent to the globe just posterior to the muscle insertions and weakly adherent in the intervening quadrants. The medial check ligament (MC) and lateral check ligament (LC) are noted. These are extensions from the sleeves of fascia surrounding these respective muscles that serve to secure them to the periorbita. Representative of the septa that encircle the anterior orbit in spoke-like fashion, strands of connective tissue are noted emanating from the inferior oblique muscle (*) to insert into the periorbita.

[1]Koornneef, L. (1977a): New insights in the human orbital connective tissue: Results of a new anatomic approach. *Arch. Ophthalmol.*, 95:1269.
Koornneef, L. (1977b): Details of the orbital connective tissue system in the adult. *Acta Morphol. Neerl. Scand.*, 15:1.
Koornneef, L. (1979): Orbital septa: Anatomy and function. *Ophthalmology*, 86:876.
Koornneef, L. (1982): Orbital connective tissue. In: *Bromedical Foundations of Ophthalmology, Vol. 1*, edited by T. D. Duane and E. A. Jaeger, Chapter 32. Harper and Row, Philadelphia.

EXTRAOCULAR MUSCLES

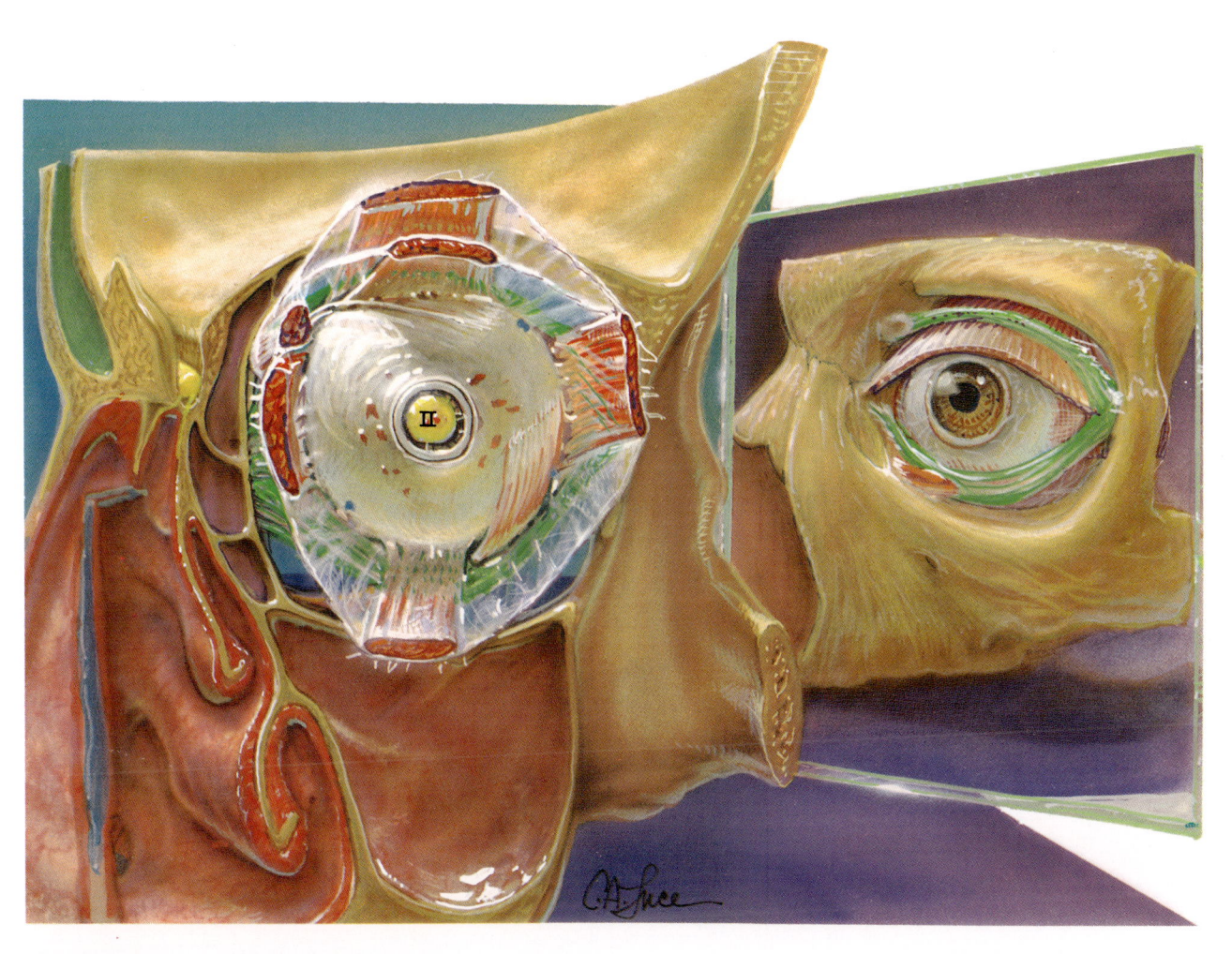

FIG. 8-4. More posteriorly, the intervening intramuscular septa are thinner and may become discontinuous, thus opening the muscle cone. Tenon's capsule continues posteriorly adherent to the globe to eventually encircle the optic nerve (II), which penetrates it. More anteriorly as the intermuscular septa thickens, the connective mass between the inferior oblique and inferior rectus muscles forms the inferior suspensory ligament of Lockwood *(green)*. Similarly, a thickening or condensation of fascia may be noted superiorly overlying or surrounding the levator muscle, i.e., Whitnall's ligament.

CHAPTER 8

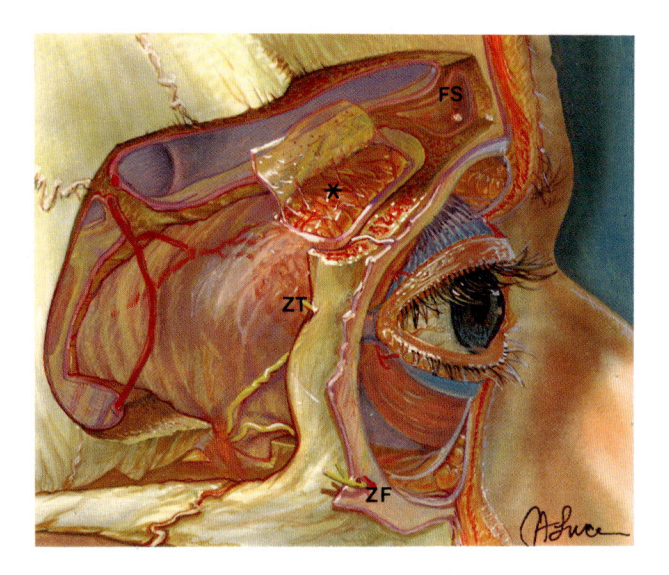

FIG. 8-5. Lateral dissection. The temporal bone and superior orbital rim are removed to expose the lateral periorbita. A periorbital flap has been elevated to expose the orbital portion of the lacrimal gland (*). An extension of the frontal sinus (FS) is noted superiorly. The zygomaticofacial and zygomaticotemporal nerves may be seen prior to exit via their respective foramina (zf, zt).

FIG. 8-6. The remaining lateral orbital rim and a portion of the periorbita have been removed, demonstrating an important anatomic landmark, i.e., the lateral rectus muscle *(arrow)* covered by a thin layer of muscular fascia. Note the lacrimal nerve and lacrimal artery coursing forward. This artery later divides into the superior and inferior lateral palpebral arteries, as noted previously. Intraconal fat (F) may be seen within the thinned intermuscular membrane.

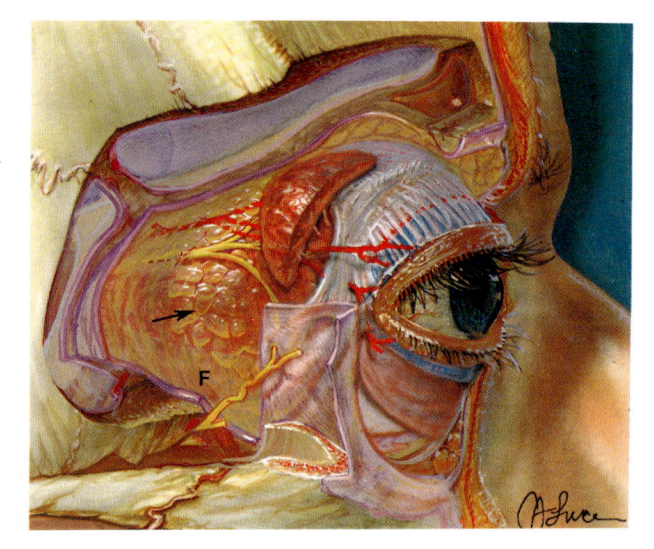

64

EXTRAOCULAR MUSCLES

FIG. 8-7. Note the lateral check ligament *(arrow)* as it arises from the lateral rectus muscle (LR). The lateral check ligament inserts into the lateral retinaculum, which is held in both forceps. The large orbital portion of the lacrimal gland (LG) is noted, as well as the lacrimal nerve (L.N.), entering the gland posteriorly.

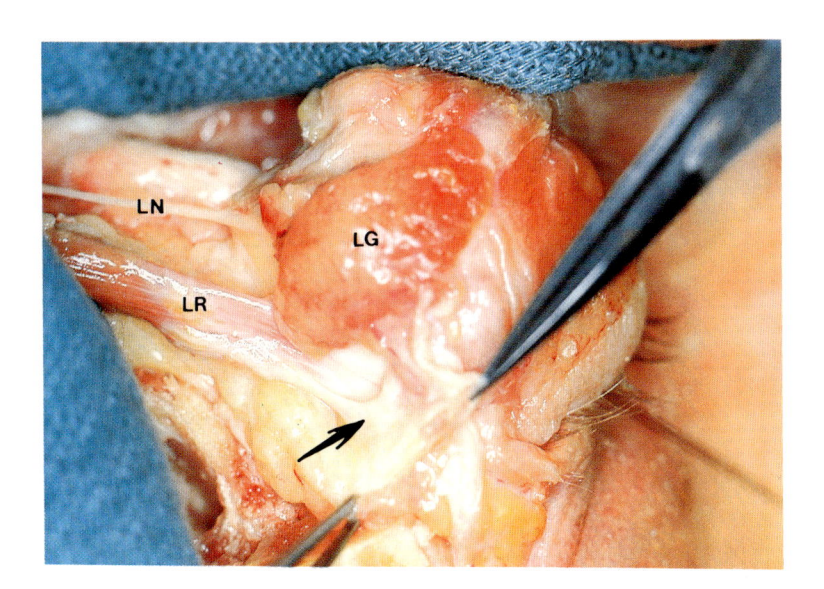

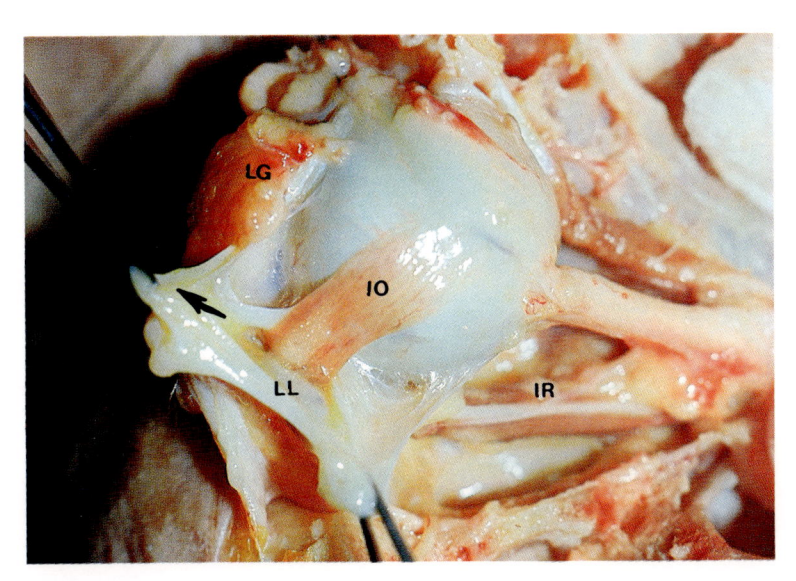

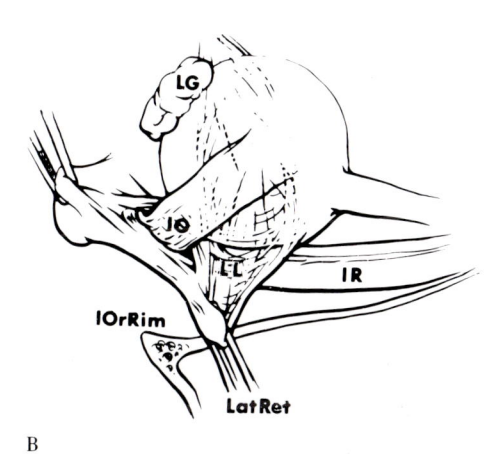

FIG. 8-8. A & B. The thickened intermuscular fascia forms a hammock anteriorly that serves to help support the globe. This suspensory ligament of Lockwood (LL) is noted beneath the globe. The inferior oblique muscle (IO) is noted piercing the intermuscular septa prior to its insertion on the globe. The lower forceps grasps the insertion of Lockwood's ligament into the lateral retinacular complex, while the upper forceps holds the insertion of the lateral canthal tendon into that same structure. The forceps are shown spread apart for demonstration only. The lacrimal gland (LG) is noted, as well as the lateral horn of the levator muscle, which splits the gland prior to insertion into the lateral retinaculum *(arrow)*. The inferior rectus muscle (IR) and the nerve to the inferior oblique muscle running with it are also depicted.

65

9

Intracranial Dissection

The orbital surgeon will frequently work in conjunction with a neurosurgeon. This relationship may be required for the extirpation of tumors, optic nerve decompression, and the management of craniofacial anomalies and traumatic deformation. Pertinent intracranial anatomy must be mastered to approach these problems with confidence. The relative positions of neurovascular structures in the middle cranial fossa to each other and to their bony habitat may provide critical clues to the surgeon about to embark on such procedures.

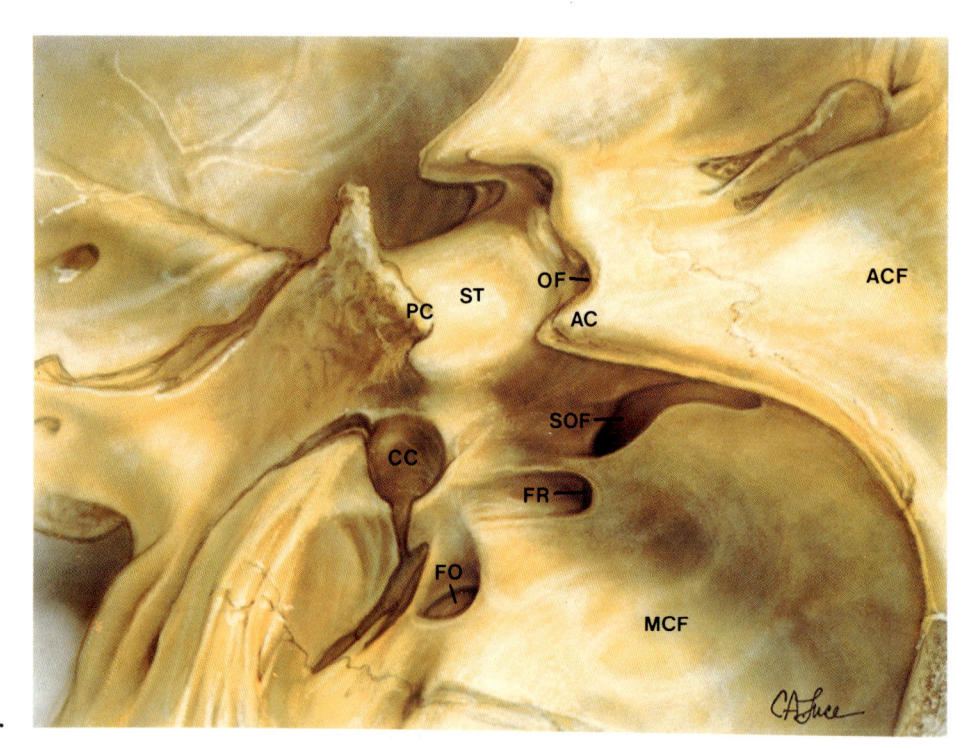

FIG. 9-1.

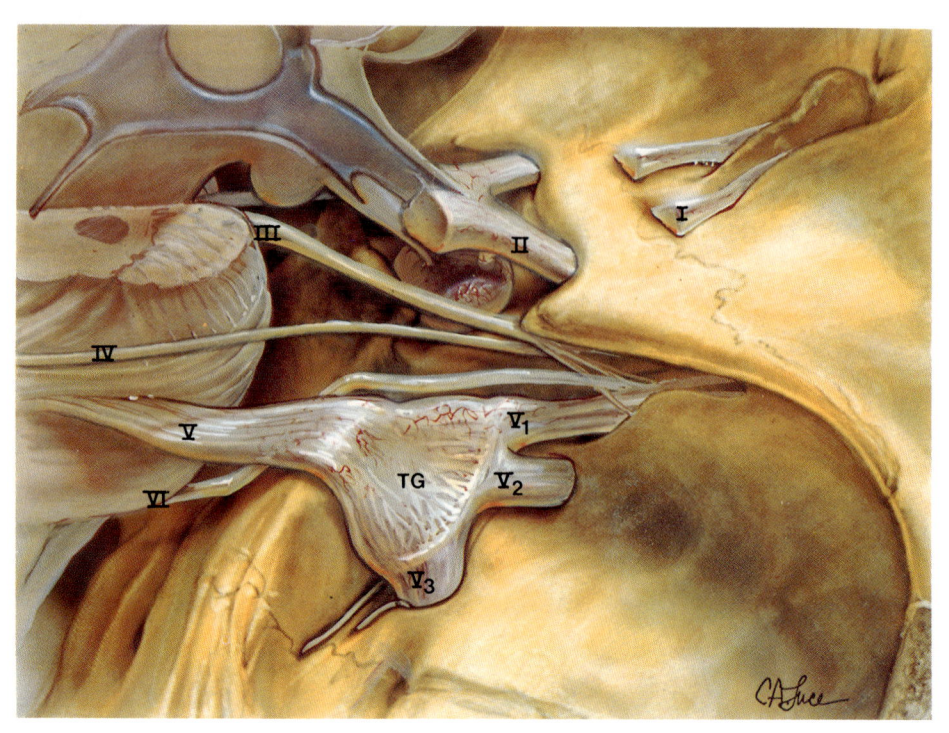

FIG. 9-2. The three motor nerves to the orbit pass through the middle cranial fossa in the cavernous sinus. These cranial nerves, specifically III, IV, and VI, are so closely grouped together that vascular, tumorous, or inflammatory conditions located in the region of the internal carotid artery or hypophysis often affect these nerves.

The oculomotor nerve (III) is noted beneath the anterior clinoid (AC) process. The trochlear nerve (IV) originates from the dorsum of the brain stem and has the longest intracranial course. The trigeminal nerve (V) separates into three divisions distal to the trigiminal ganglion (TG). The ophthalmic division (V$_1$) runs through the lateral wall of the cavernous sinus, divides into three branches, and enters the orbit via the superior orbital fissure. The maxillary division (V$_2$) runs along the lower lateral wall of the cavernous sinus to exit via the foramen rotundum (FR). The mandibular division (V$_3$) passes through the foramen ovale (FO). The abducens nerve (VI) enters the cavernous sinus inferiorly via an intradural course from the posterior cranial fossa.

INTRACRANIAL DISSECTION

FIG. 9-1. The optic foramen (OF) transmits the ophthalmic artery and the optic nerve. The maxillary division of the trigeminal nerve (V₂) enters the foramen rotundum (FR). Most other pertinent structures go through the superior orbital fissure (SOF). The carotid canal (CC) and foramen ovale (FO) are noted, through which the internal carotid artery and V₃, the mandibular division of the trigeminal, pass, respectively. The anterior clinoid (Ac) and posterior clinoid (Pc) processes surround the sella turcica (Se), or seat for the pituitary gland. The middle cranial fossa (MCF) and anterior cranial fossa (ACF) are noted.

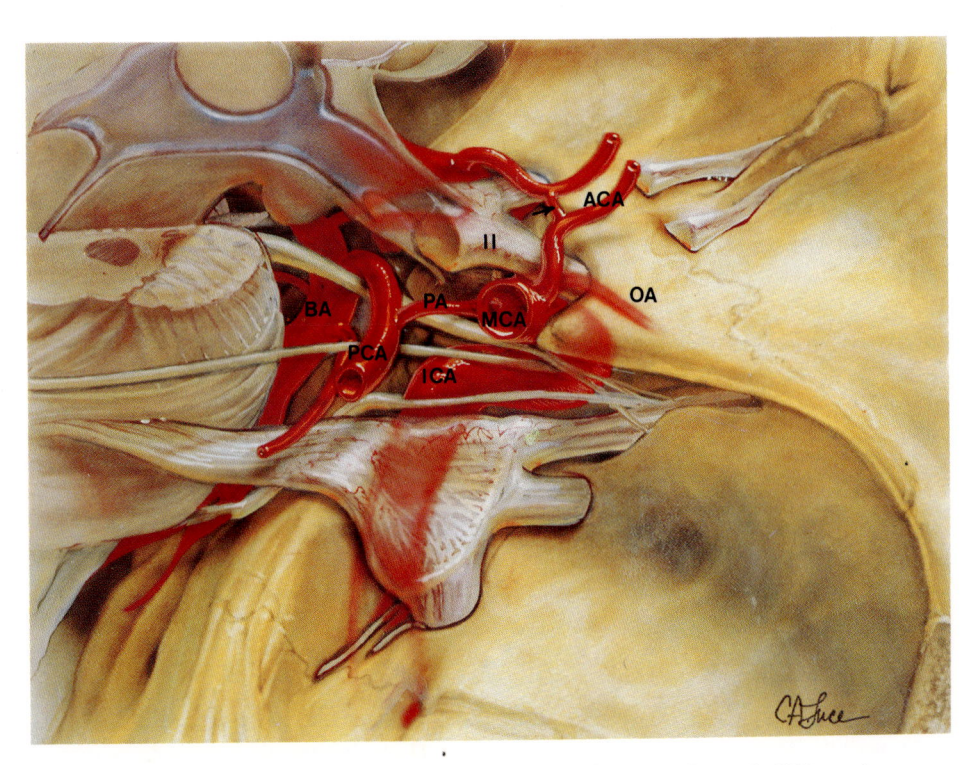

FIG. 9-3. The internal carotid artery (ICA) enters the skull through the carotid canal (CC) in the petrous portion of the temporal bone. The artery then follows the canal medially and anteriorly to pierce the dura as it turns upward to lie within the caverous sinus.

The first major intracranial branch of the internal carotid artery is the ophthalmic artery (OA), arising just posterior to the optic canal. The ophthalmic artery enters the optic canal inferior to the optic nerve (II) but within the dural sheath surrounding the nerve.

The carotid then courses upward to divide into the two terminal branches, the anterior cerebral artery (ACA) and middle cerebral artery (MCA). The anterior cerebral arteries connect via the anterior communicating artery *(arrow)*. Just prior to this division, the posterior communicating artery arises (PA) and joins the posterior cerebral artery (PCA). The circle of Willis is composed of these three vessels.

CHAPTER 9

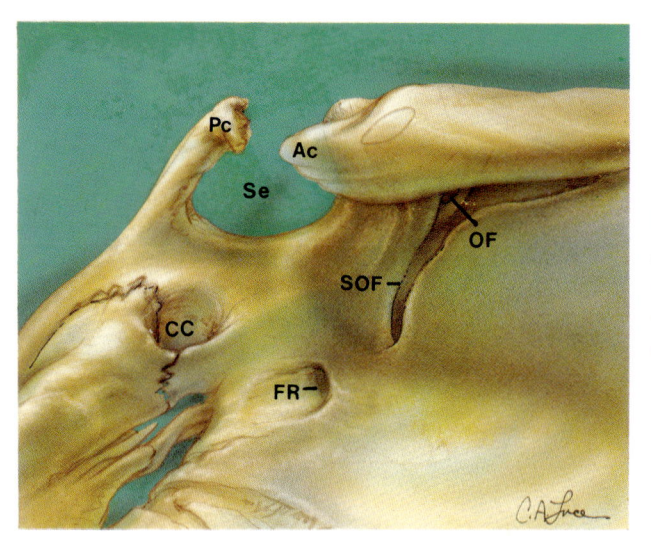

FIG. 9-4. A: Lateral closeup of skull base behind orbit. *Note:* sella turcica (Se); superior orbital fissure (SOF); foramen rotundum (FR); carotid canal (CC); anterior clinoid process (Ac); posterior clinoid process (Pc); and optic foramen exit (OF); note the ghosted outline of the optic canal.

FIG. 9-4. B: The dura *(pink)* lines the cranial vault. A separation between two leaves of dura at the sphenoid body forms the cavernous sinus *(blue)*. The cavernous sinus communicates with the ophthalmic veins, central retinal vein, middle and inferior cerebral veins, and middle meningeal veins, as well as the pyterygoid plexus and superior and inferior petrosal sinuses. The pituitary gland (PG), which lies medial to the cavernous sinus, as well as the optic nerve (II) are noted.

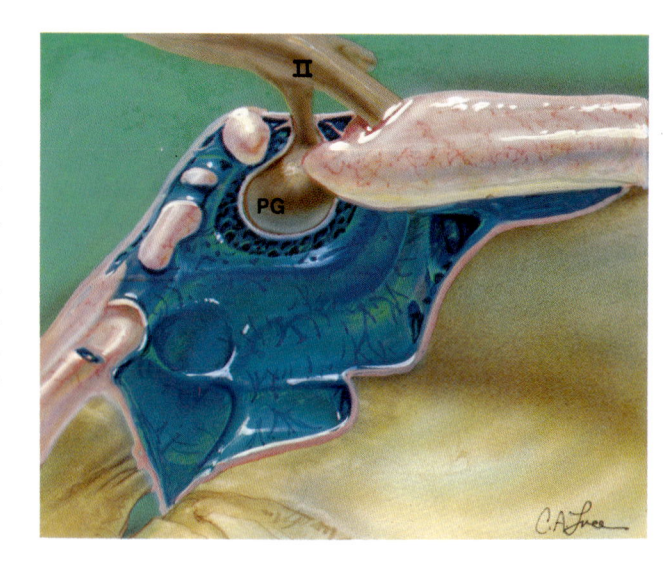

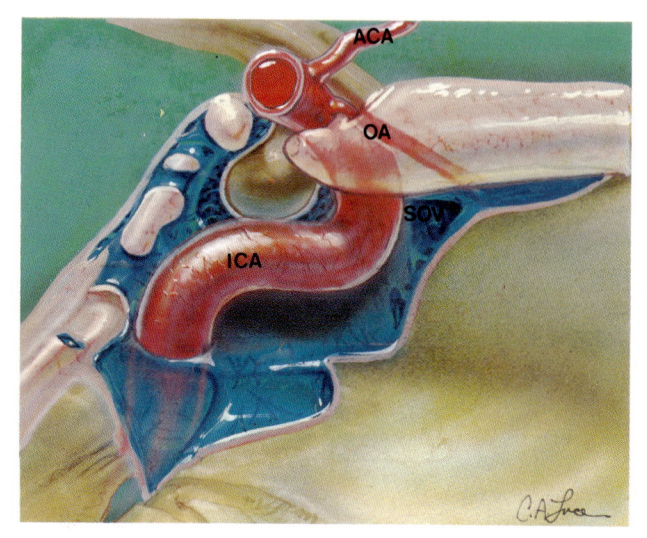

FIG. 9-4. C: The intracavernous portion of the internal carotid artery (ICA) forms an "S" curve. The first branch, the ophthalmic artery (OA), is noted as well as the anterior cerebral artery (ACA).

INTRACRANIAL DISSECTION

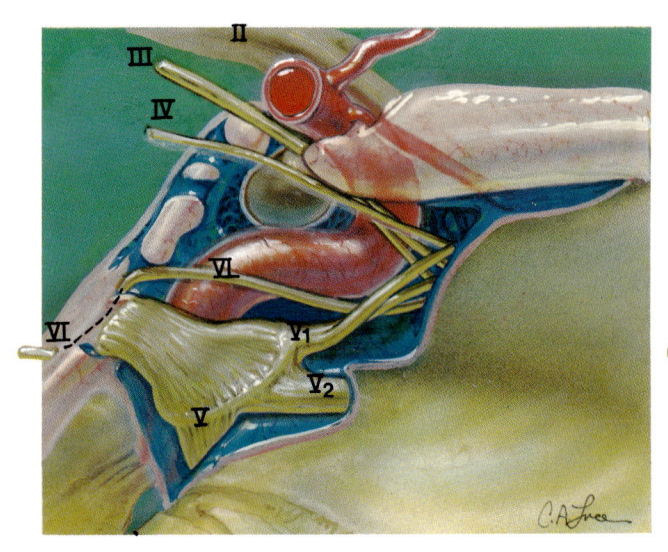

FIG. 9-4. D: In the inferior portion of the cavernous sinus, the maxillary division of the trigeminal nerve (V₂) exits via the foramen rotundum. The ophthalmic division (V₁) passes upward to enter the superior orbital fissure. The abducens nerve (VI) is closely adherent to the lateral portion of the internal carotid artery. In the posterior portion of the cavernous sinus, the oculomotor nerve (III) lies superior to the smaller trochlear nerve (IV). As stated previously, the oculomotor nerve enters the orbit within the annulus, but the trochlear nerve enters above the annulus.

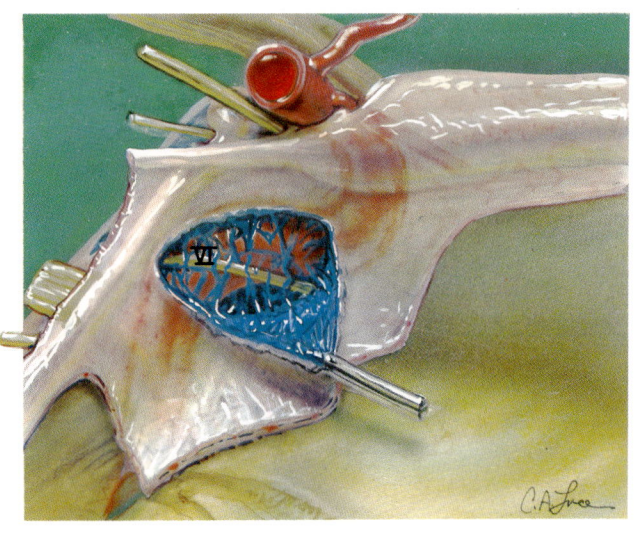

FIG. 9-4. E: The lateral wall of the cavernous sinus is replaced. Actually, this lateral wall consists of a thicker outer layer and a less dense inner layer. The inner layer surrounds the oculomotor, trochlear, ophthalmic, and maxillary nerves. Note the abducens nerve (VI) lateral to the internal carotid artery.

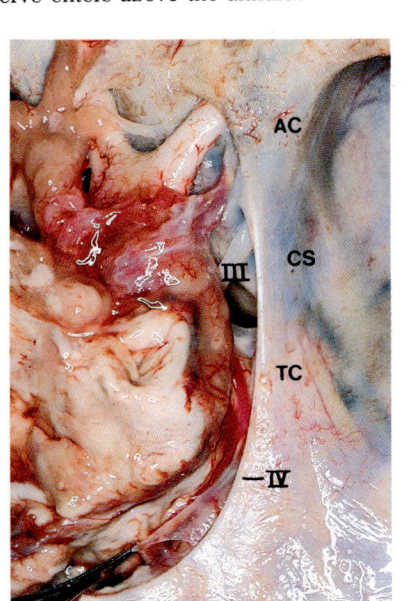

FIG. 9-5. The free margin of the tentorium cerebri (TC) extends back from the anterior clinoid process (AC). The oculomotor nerve (III) proceeds laterally to pierce the dura and traverse the lateral wall of the cavernous sinus (CS). Barely visible, the trochlear nerve (IV) lies near the lower surface of the tentorium to enter the dural shelf.

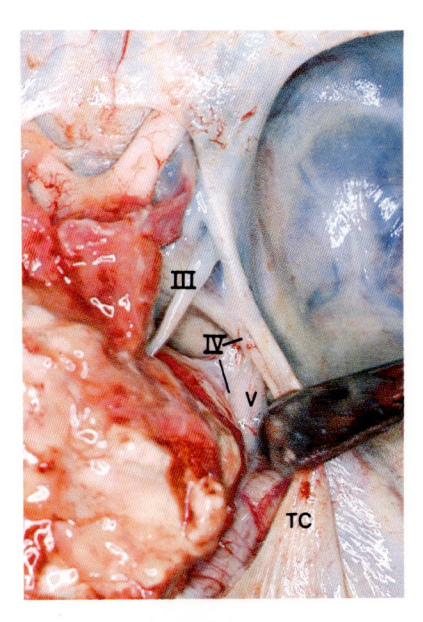

FIG. 9-6. Lateral retraction of the tentorium cerebri (TC) reveals the trochlear nerve (IV) entering the dura just below the free margin. It then travels within the cavernous sinus. The oculomotor nerve (III) is again noted, as well as the root of the trigeminal nerve (V) crossing over the petrous ridge.

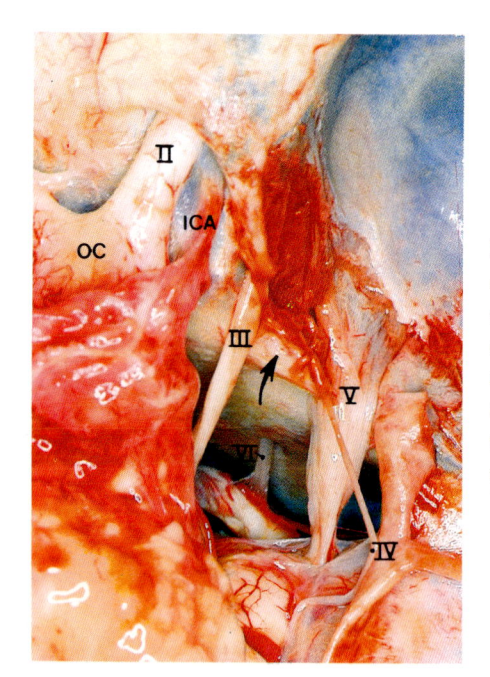

FIG. 9-7. The optic chiasm (OC) is viewed from behind. The optic nerve (II) enters its optic canal superomedial to the internal carotid artery (ICA). The margin of the tentorium cerebri has been removed to expose the inside of the cavernous sinus. The oculomotor nerve (III) passes over the petroclinoid ligament *(arrow)*, entering the dural wall of the cavernous sinus. The trochlear nerve (IV) is visible because the free margin of the tentorium has been removed to expose it. The relative positions of the trigeminal (V) and abducens nerves (VI) are noted.

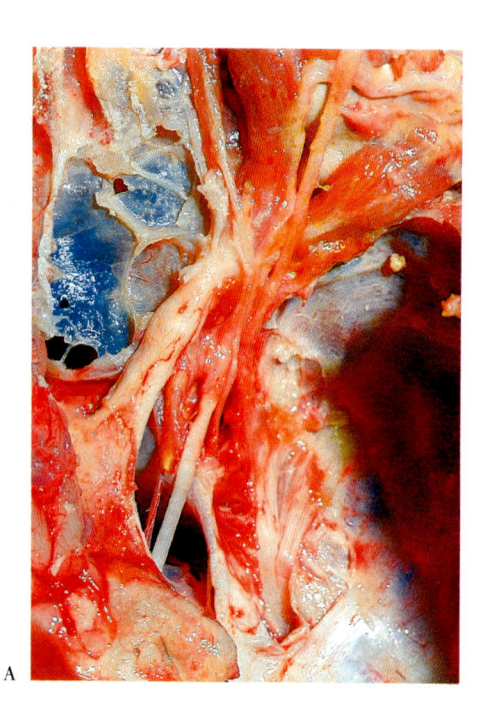

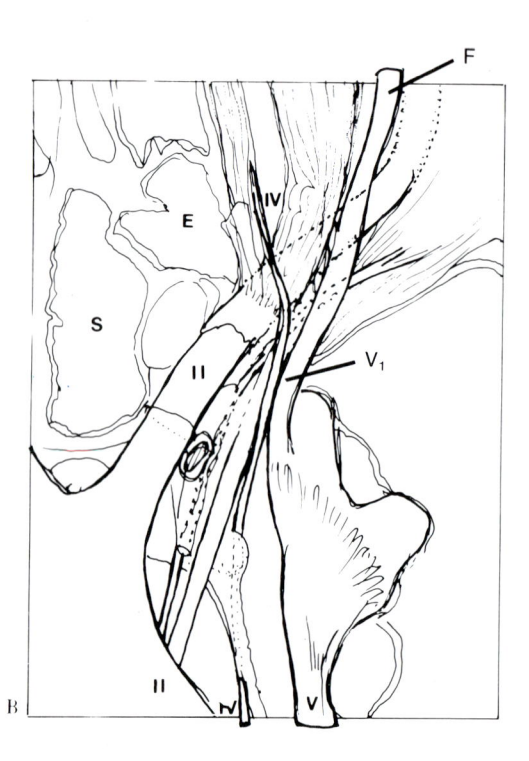

FIG. 9-8. A & B. The roof of the orbit has been removed in continuity with the superior orbital fissure. The roof of the optic canal and bony coverings of the adjacent sinuses have also been excised. The sphenoid sinus mucosa (S) and ethmoid sinus mucosa (E) have been left intact. Note the close relationship of the optic nerve (II) to the posterior lateral walls of these sinuses. The optic nerve courses through the optic canal within the lesser wing of the sphenoid for approximately 10 mm to enter the orbit.

The cavernous sinus has been unroofed, exposing the nerves that lie within it. The oculomotor nerve (III) divides into its upper and lower divisions within the cavernous sinus to enter the orbit within the annulus via the superior orbital fissure. The trochlear nerve (IV) first courses laterally to the oculomotor nerve within the cavernous sinus, then crosses superomedially above the oculomotor nerve. The trochlear nerve enters the orbit through the superior orbital fissure above the annulus to innervate the superior oblique muscle (SO). The ophthalmic division of the trigeminal (V_1) divides within the cavernous sinus prior to entering the fissure. Note the frontal branch (F) of the ophthalmic division.

Subject Index

A
Abducens nerve
  course, 68
  extraocular muscle supply, 60
  and internal carotid artery, 71
  in oculomotor foramen, 60
  and oculomotor nerve, 57
  and trigeminal nerve, 72
Alveolar nerves, 4,32
Ampulla of the canaliculus, 36–37
Angular infraorbital artery, 28
Annulus of Zinn, 8,60
Anterior cerebral artery, 69–70
Anterior ciliary arteries, 60
Anterior clinoid process, 68–71
Anterior communicating artery, 69
Anterior cranial fossa, 54,69
Anterior deep temporal nerve, 18
Anterior ethmoidal air cells, 9,55
Anterior ethmoidal artery, 4
Anterior ethmoidal foramen, 4,54
Anterior ethmoidal nerve, 12,54
Anterior lacrimal crest, 4,25,36,42
Anterior maxilla, 19,32
Anterior superior alveolar nerve, 4,12,32
Anterior tarsus, 26
Arcus marginalis, 25,28–29

B
Basic lacrimal secretors, 35
Bulbar fascia, 30

C
Canaliculus, 36–37
Canthral angle, 36
Capsulopalpebral fascia, 28,30
Capsulopalpebral head, 30
Carotid canal, 69–70
Caruncle, 36
Cavernous sinus, 70–72
Central fat pad, 25,27
Central retinal artery, 11
Cheek, 13–19
Cheek ligament, lateral rectus muscle, 49–50
Cheek muscle, 19
Ciliary ganglion, 56
Circle of Willis, 69
Common tendinous ring, 60
Conjunctival fornix, 30
Conjunctival lining, 23
Conjunctival mucin-secreting cells, 35
Cornea, tear system, 35
Corrugator muscle, 14–15, 24
Cranial nerve III, 8,68
Cranial nerve IV, 68
Cranial nerve V, 8,12

Cranial nerve VI, 8,68
Cranial vault, 70
Cribriform plate, 52,56
  crista galli, 9,56
  "nasal slit,", 54
Crista galli, 9,52,56

D
Deep temporal fascia, 17
Depressor supercilii fibers, 42
Dorsal nasal nerve, 12

E
Ethmoid bone, 2,4
Ethmoid labyrinth, 46
Ethmoid sinus, 56
Ethmoid sinus mucosa, 72
Ethmoidal ostia, 9
  and nasofrontal duct, 39
External carotid artery, 10
External nasal nerve, 12
Extraocular muscles, 59–65
  functions, 60
Eyelids, 21–32

F
Facial nerve, 16,28
Fascia bulbi, 62
Fascial bone periosteum, 25
Fascial framework, 62–65
Foramen ovale, 9, 68–69
Foramen rotundum, 4,8–9,68–71
Foramen spinosum, 9
Forehead, 13–19
Frontal bone, 2,4,6–7,9,24,52
Frontal nerve, 8,12,53,60
Frontal sinus, 9,52,64
Frontalis muscle, 14–18
Frontoethmoidal suture, 4
Frontosphenoidal sutures, 9

G
Galeal aponeurosis, 14,16
Gillies maneuver, 17
Glabella, 7

H
Hasner's valve, 38
Horner's muscle, 23,42

I
Inferior meatus, 37
Inferior oblique muscle
  and eyelids, 23,31
  functions, 60

  and intermuscular septa, 65
  and Lockwood's ligament, 63
  oculomotor nerve, 57, 60
  origin, 4,30,60
Inferior ophthalmic vein, 4
Inferior orbital fissure, 4,8
Inferior orbital margin, 4
Inferior orbital rim, 25
Inferior palpebral muscle, 30
Inferior rectus muscle, 65
  capsulopalpebral fascia, 28
  and common tendinous ring, 60
  course of, 57
  and eyelids, 23
  functions, 60
  and inferior oblique muscle, 30
  and Lockwood's ligament, 63
  and oculomotor nerve, 57,60
Inferior suspensory ligament, 49,63
  lateral anterior portion, 50
Inferior transverse suspensory ligament, 23
Inferior turbinate, 32,38
Inferolateral orbital rim, 28
Infraorbital artery, 4
Infraorbital foramen, 4,7,28,31
Infraorbital groove, 4
Infraorbital nerve, 4,12,31
  branches, 19
  and superior alveolar nerve, 32
  and tear system, 38
Infratemporal fossa, 4
Infratrochlear artery, 28
Infratrochlear nerve, 12,54
Interglandular fascia, 49,65
Intermuscular septa, 62–63,65
Internal carotid artery
  and abducens nerve, 71
  in carotid canal, 69
  course of, 69
  intracavernous portion, 70
  ophthalmic artery origin, 53,69
  and optic nerve, 72
  orbit relationship, 10–11
  "S" curve, 70
Internal maxillary artery, 10
Intracranial dissection, 67–72

K
Krause's glands, 35

L
Lacrimal apparatus, 33–39
Lacrimal artery, 24,28,64
Lacrimal bone, 2,4,6
Lacrimal diaphragm, 37
Lacrimal drainage system, 34
Lacrimal exocrine glands, 35
Lacrimal fascia, 36

Subject Index

Lacrimal fossa
   and lacrimal sac, 4,36,44
   and middle turbinate, 39
Lacrimal gland, 26–27,55
   basic secretors, 35
   divisions, 35,49
   inferolateral pole, 49
   and lacrimal fossa, 4
   and lateral rectus muscle, 50
   orbital portion, 64–65
Lacrimal lake, 37
Lacrimal nerve, 12
   and the annulus, 8
   course of, 53,60,64–65
Lacrimal pump, 37
Lacrimal sac, 4,36–37
   height, 37
   and medial canthal tendon, 44
   and orbicularis oculi fibers, 42
Lacrimal secretory system, 35
Lamina papyracea, 4,46
   and ethmoid labyrinth, 46
Lateral canthal tendon, 48–49,65
   and orbital system, 25,48
   splitting of, 48
Lateral cheek ligament, 62,65
Lateral oblique right orbit, 2
Lateral orbital rim, 48
Lateral orbital tubercle, 48
Lateral orbital wall, 52,57
Lateral rectus muscle, 57,64
   abducens nerve, 60
   as anatomical landmark, 64
   cheek ligament of, 49
   function, 60
   and lacrimal gland, 50
   and lacrimal nerve, 53
   and lateral cheek ligament, 65
   motor nerve, 57
   origin of, 60
   and superior orbital fissure, 8
Lateral retinaculum, 30,47–50,65
Lateral wall, 4
Levator anguli oris, 19
Levator aponeurosis, 23,26–27
   lateral horn, 49
Levator labii superioris, 19
Levator muscle
   aponeurosis, 23,26–27
   and infraorbital nerve branches, 19
   lateral horn, 65
   Muller's muscle origin, 23,27
   oculomotor nerve, 55,60
   origin, 23,27,60
   Whitnall's nerve, 26,63
Levator of nasal ala, 19
Levator palpebrae muscle
   course of, 54
   and eyelids, 23
   and frontal nerve, 53
   and superior rectus muscle, 55
Levator palpebrae superioris muscle, 24,26

lacrimal gland division, 35
Ligament of Lockwood, 23,30,49–50
Limbal mucin-secreting cells, 35
Lockwood's ligament, 23,30,49–50,63,65
Luschka's nerve, 54

M

Marginal artery, 23
Masseter muscle, 18
Maxilla, 2,4,7,19,29–30,32
   and medial canthal tendon, 42
Maxillary sinus mucosa, 31,38
Maxillary sinuses, 9
Medial canthal tendon
   anterior portion, 14
   and canaliculi, 36
   and lacrimal sac, 37
   and orbicularis oculi, 24,28,42
   release of, dystopia, 45
   vertical fascial expansion, 44
Medial canthus, 41–46
Medial cheek ligament, 62
Medial fat pad, 25
Medial orbicularis muscle, 42
Medial orbit, 36
Medial orbital margin, 42
Medial orbital wall, 4,52
Medial palpebral arterial vessels, 25
Medial rectus muscle, 56–57
   anterior ethmoidal nerve, 54
   function, 60
   and oculomotor nerve, 56–57, 60
   and optic nerve, 60
   and superior oblique muscle, 56
Meibomian glands, 32,35
Meningeal foramen, 4
Middle cerebral artery, 69
Middle cranial fossa, 8,9,68–69
Middle meatus, 39
Middle meningeal artery, 4,8,10
Middle superior alveolar nerves, 4
Midline crista galli, 52
Moll's glands, 35
Muller's muscle, 23,26–27

N

Nasal fat compartment, 27
Nasal nerve, 54
"Nasal slit," 54
Nasalis transversus, 19
Nasociliary nerve, 12,53–54,56–57
   course of, 54,56
   in oculomotor foramen, 8,60
   and superior oblique muscle, 54,56
Nasofrontal ducts, 9,39,52
Nasofrontal suture, 46
Nasolabial fold, 31
Nasolacrimal canals, 9
Nasolacrimal duct, 32
   and inferior oblique muscle, 30
   intraosseous portion, 37
   tear system, 37–38

O

Oculomotor foramen, 8,60
Oculomotor nerve
   and anterior clinoid process, 68
   in cavernous sinus, 71–72
   course of, 57
   extraocular muscle supply, 60
   inferior division, 56–57,60
   in oculomotor foramen, 60
   and petroclinoid ligament, 72
   superior division, 55–56,60
Olfactory bulb, 56
Olfactory nerve, 56
Ophthalmic artery, 11
   branches of, 11
   extraocular muscle supply, 60
   intracavernous portion, 70
   in muscle cone, 11
   in optic foramen, 69
   origin and course, 53,69
Ophthalmic veins, 8,60
Optic canal, 4,7,52,72
Optic chiasm, 72
Optic foramen, 4,9,69–70
Optic foramen exit, 70
Optic nerve, 53,57,72
   and cavernous sinus, 70
   course of, 56,60
   coverings of, 53
   and frontal sinus, 52
   intracranial length, 53
   and optic canal, 72
   in optic foramen, 69
   and Tenon's capsule, 63
Orbicularis oculi muscle, 23–26
   blood supply, 28
   divisions, 24
   and eyelids, 23–26,42
   lacrimal sac relationship, 42
   and levator muscle, 19
   and medial canthus, 14,42
   oblique extension, 19
Orbital axis, 7
Orbital depth, 6
Orbital dissection, 51–57
Orbital fat, 23,42
Orbital floor, 4,29,31
Orbital height, 6
Orbital margin, 25,29
Orbital roof, 4,52
Orbital septum, 23,25–26,28–29,42
   and lateral canthal tendon, 48
Orbital walls, 4,9

P

Palatine bone, 2,4
Palpebral lacrimal glands, 35,49
Palpebral orbicularis oculi muscle, 24
   components, 42
   divisions, 24
   and medial canthal tendon, 42
Papilla, 36

Subject Index

Parotid lymph nodes, 28
Pars lacrimalis, 42
Periorbita, 25,28,48–49,52,55
Periosteum, 60
Peripheral arterial arcade, 23
Petroclinoid ligament, 72
Petrous ridge, 71
Pituitary gland, 70
Posterior cerebral artery, 69
Posterior clinoid process, 69–70
Posterior communicating artery, 69
Posterior cranial fossa, 68
Posterior ethmoidal air cells, 9
Posterior ethmoidal artery, 4
Posterior ethmoidal foramen, 4,54
Posterior ethmoidal nerve, 12,54
Posterior lacrimal crest, 4,25,36,44
Posterior superior alveolar nerve, 12
Preauricular lymph nodes, 28
Precorneal tear film, 34–35
Preseptal orbicularis oculi muscle, 24,37,44
Preseptal palpebral orbicularis oculi muscle, 42
Pretarsal orbicularis oculi muscle, 24,36–37
Pretarsal palpebral orbicularis oculi muscle, 42
Pretarsal space, 23
Procerus muscles, 14
Pterygopalatine fossa, 4
Puncti, eyelids, 36–37

R
Recess of Eisler, 25
Reflex lacrimal secretors, 35
Retrobulbar neuritis, 60

S
Sella turcica, 69–70
Semilunar fold, 36
Sensory nerves, 12
Sphenoethmoid recesses, 9
Sphenoid bone, 4
Sphenoid greater wing, 2,7
Sphenoid lesser wing, 2
   levator palpebrae muscle, 54
   and optic canal, 52
   and optic foramen, 9
   optic nerve course, 60,72
   and orbital wall, 4
   superior orbital fissure, 7
Sphenoid sinus, 9,56
Sphenoid sinus mucosa, 72

Sphenopalatine ganglion, 4
Submandibular regional lymph nodes, 28
Subperiosteal dissection, 6
Superficial temporal artery, 10,15
Superficial temporal fascia, 16–18
Superficial temporal vessels, 17
Superior lateral conjunctival fornix, 35
Superior oblique muscle, 27
   anterior oblique nerve, 54
   functions, 60
   and medial rectus muscle, 56
   and nasociliary nerve, 54,46
   at orbital apex, 55
   origin, 60
   post-trochlear portion, 55
   and superior rectus muscle, 55
   and trochlear fossa tendon, 4
   and trochlear nerve (IV), 53,56,60,72
Superior oblique tendon, 25, 27, 30
Superior oblique trochlear pulley, 25
Superior orbital fissure, 8, 69–70
   length of, 8
   and meningeal foramen, 4
   nasociliary nerve, 54
   and sphenoid bone, 7
   trigeminal nerve, 53,68,71
   trochlear nerve, 53
Superior orbital rim, 7,64
Superior rectus muscle, 54
   and common tendinous ring, 60
   and eyelids, 23,27
   functions, 60
   oculomotor nerve, 55–56,60
   and superior oblique muscle, 55
Superior temporal line, 17
Superior transverse ligament of Whitnall, see Whitnall's ligament
Superomedial orbital margin, 4,24
Supraciliary arches, 7
Supraorbital bony bar, 55
Supraorbital foramen, 7,25
Supraorbital nerve, 12,14–15,53
Supraorbital notch, 7,26
Supraorbital vessels, 15
Supratrochlear nerve, 12,53
Suspensory ligament of Lockwood, 23,30,49–50,63,65
Sympathetic nerve fibers, 8

T
Tarsal mucin-secreting cells, 35
Tarsal plates, 27,32
   height of, 32
Tarsus, 23,26,30,32
Tear ducts, 35

Temporal bone, 64
Temporal fascia, 17–18,28
Temporal fossa, 6,18
Temporal region, 13–19
Temporalis muscle, 16–18
Tenon's capsule, 62–63
Tensor tarsi, 42
Tentorium cerebri, 71–72
Transverse facial vessels, 28
Trigeminal ganglion, 12,68
Trigeminal nerve, mandibular division, 12,68
Trigeminal nerve, maxillary division, 4,12,68–69,71
Trigeminal nerve, ophthalmic division, 12,53,68,71–72
   frontal branch, 72
Trochlea, 26,55
Trochlear fossa, 4
Trochlear nerve (IV), 8,60
   and annulus of Zinn, 8
   in cavernous sinus, 71
   course and divisions, 53,68,72
   extraocular muscle supply, 60
   and frontal nerve, 53
   and superior oblique muscle, 56,72
   and tentorium cerebri, 71–72

V
Visual axis, 7

W
Whitnall's ligament
   lateral portion, 49
   and levator muscle, 23,25,63
   medial component, 55
   and superior rectus muscle, 55
Whitnall's tubercle, 4,48
Wolffring's glands, 35

Z
Zeis's glands, 35
Zygoma, 2,6,7,16,18
Zygomatic arch, 16–17
Zygomatic bone, 4,6,18
Zygomatic minor, 19
Zygomatic nerve, 4,12,28
Zygomaticofacial nerve, 4,6,12,18,64
Zygomaticofacial vessels, 28
Zygomaticofrontal suture, 6–7
Zygomaticotemporal nerve, 4,12,18,64
Zygomaticus major, 19
Zygomatomaxillary suture, 7